A Poi   ...c -
A Nourished Soul

Toxic Mixes, Psychic Fixes

A Poisoned Life -
A Nourished Soul

Toxic Mixes, Psychic Fixes

Brian Hopkinson

Published by Tiger Script

A POISONED LIFE – A NOURISHED SOUL

A Tiger Script book
First published in Great Britain 2022
Copyright © Brian Hopkinson
All rights reserved

Tiger Script
Manchester, Great Britain

Cover design by Deeper Blue www.wearedeeper.blue
ISBN: 978-1-9160819-6-3

Dedication

Thanks to my sister Verna and brother Stuart, my nieces Melanie, Rebecca and Phillipa, my nephew Shane, and all the family members who have helped me along the way.

To chemical victims I came to know only by phone, now sadly deceased: Geoff Lewis, Hazel Staddon and Lorraine Taylor.

To mora therapist Karen Barlow for her friendly and invaluable help.

To Emily Doherty, a special soul.

To Georgina Alexandra, a good friend.

To Annabelle Jane Rhodes, a free spirit.

To Louise Ellis, a fighter for the cause.

And of course to my partner for thirty-four years, Eileen.

For all sufferers of ME–CFS who endure the added injury of not being believed by the mainstream medical establishment—keep the faith, find alternatives. Simple changes made a big difference for me, such as filtering my drinking water, eating an organic diet, regularly using reiki treatments and mora therapy, and avoiding chemicals as much as possible.

CONTENTS

INTRODUCTION

I've always had a forthright manner and a strong sense of what is right and wrong. Even as a child I would always speak out against what I deemed to be injustices. Which is why I developed an affinity with so-called radicals in society such as songwriters John Lennon and Bob Dylan, President Nelson Mandela, environmentalist Rachel Carson, and even the miners' leader Arthur Scargill. These were remarkable people who were willing to speak out about others who suffered oppressions, and in some cases were prepared to do something about it.

This strong sense of injustice in my character has played a major role in keeping me fighting for so long against cynicism, prejudice, ignorance, and at times downright arrogance from medics, councillors, government officials and people purporting to represent victims of ME–CFS and chemically damaged victims.

My personal battle with myalgic encephalomyelitis (ME) and chronic fatigue syndrome (CFS), and subsequent clashes with the medical profession, have prompted me to write this book in an attempt to encourage the majority of the medical profession to stop treating people with ME–CFS with disrespect. As far back as 1969 the World Health Organisation documented ME–CFS as a neurological condition, so why does the UK medical establishment find it so hard to accept? It is estimated that an astonishing 250,000 people in the UK have ME–CFS symptoms, 25% of whom are bedridden. Many face cruel, lonely deaths—on average one sufferer per week commits suicide.

Common symptoms of ME–CFS include:
- sleep irregularities
- muscle/joint pain
- headaches
- sore throat
- difficulty remembering or concentrating
- flu-like symptoms
- dizziness or sickness
- heart palpitations

After six months the symptoms often worsen, and include...
- Unrelenting fatigue
- Isolation
- Abnormal body temperature control
- Drug, alcohol and chemical intolerance
- Mood swings (due to hormonal imbalance)
- Weight loss

- Foggy brain
- Short-term memory loss

I used to wonder why there was a great reluctance by the medical establishment to even listen and try to understand how chemicals can have a devastating effect on people's lives.

Why does the mainstream medical profession refuse to accept that ME–CFS is a chemically toxic neurological disease and why do they refuse to carry out tests that would prove it? There is overwhelming evidence stretching back decades that supports what chemicals have done to me, to the planet, and to everything on it, and for a long time been swept under the carpet.

I once asked my doctor how many years it takes to qualify as a GP.

He said, 'Approximately seven.'

I then asked, 'How much of that time is given to studying neurotoxic substances and their effects?'

He replied, 'Roughly two hours.'

Need I say more?

I began reading everything I could on the subject. I was amazed to find books such as *Stop the 21st Century Killing You* by Dr Paula Baillie-Hamilton and *Detoxify or Die* by Dr Sherry Rogers (full list in the bibliography). Here were two eminently qualified doctors willing to write and speak the truth about what we've been exposed to in our daily lives for decades.

This led me to believe that there was possibly a genetic link with exposures from chemicals, and the possibility of certain diseases affecting people with a variant in their genes. After all, this link was already well established in certain inherited conditions such as Huntingdon's disease and breast cancers.

I became one of the 25% of sufferers who was either housebound or bedridden with the disease, in my case for six years. Through a monumental effort I managed to relieve the living nightmare by investigating what led to my condition (exposure to organophosphates, commonly known as OPs) before discovering the most fascinating and wonderful natural healing technique: reiki. I have no qualms in saying it rescued me from my personal living hell. In common with most ME sufferers, my body cannot tolerate conventional medication, so discovering reiki healing was a blessing from the gods.

However, it was not just what it did for me that was so life changing, it has also helped countless family members and friends in the most jaw-dropping ways.

What you are about to read is purely my opinion and perception of events. I am not medically qualified, but I would say that I am qualified as a reiki master, and most definitely qualified in suffering. What I have been through and what I continue to suffer (albeit at a more tolerable level) has taught me much about myself, and more importantly about healing the soul and spirit as well as the body.

It is heartwarming to see reiki treatments being introduced (though slowly) in hospitals. Cancer patients are now benefitting from its soothing energies and its power to detoxify following chemotherapies, thereby enhancing the feeling of well-being.

A concrete example of reiki's power can be illustrated with the occasion on which I spent ten days in hospital in 2010 with a fractured hip. I was unable to take pharmaceutical pain relief. Instead, reiki got me through. The medics were amazed, but in the end they learned very little and continued to treat me with disrespect—90% of them had never heard of ME–CFS *or* reiki, a double whammy of ignorance.

Reiki is not a cure-all, but it is a technique that will help you to change if you want to change. It works for the greatest good—for you and for everyone around you. It gave me hope when I most needed it, and overturned my feeling of being abandoned, of not being able to contribute, especially cruel in my case as I was living with a long-suffering partner with multiple sclerosis. I couldn't do half of what I wanted to do for Eileen.

But the crucial question is, What caused my ME–CFS? I believe it was exposure to environmental chemicals at work (as a groundsman during the period 1983–1992) and my proximity to farms, chemical factories and a golf course, and living next to a paper mill (only 200 metres away) for thirty years. The problem stemmed from my body's inability to detoxify (metabolise) the numerous toxic chemicals to which I was exposed, not just since my birth but also while being carried for nine months by my mother. Her history of living next to a chemical factory while pregnant—and long before that—also had an effect on my health later in life.

You may ask, Why was Brian affected and not others who lived close by? That's a fair question. You may also ask, Why do some people get the flu and not others? Because some people's immune systems are more susceptible than others. To explore that question, we shall dig a little into the body's gene responses.

Many studies and papers have been produced over the last twenty years that examine ill health associated with chemicals, which is often caused by exposure in the workplace. Some brilliant books have tried to highlight the dangers of everyday chemicals. Check out the bibliography at the back of the book for details. These books are packed with useful information on how to change the way you live with chemicals, and where to find equally good, safer alternatives.

The following is a list of doctors and scientists who have written medical reports showing my chemically induced illness.

Dr Jean Monro, *Breakspear Hospital, Hemel Hempstead*

Dr Bob Davies, *Taunton, Devon*

Dr S.K. Tamin, (*Department of Work and Pensions*)

Dr David Freed, *Manchester University (allergist)*

Dr Helen Card, *Clinical psychologist*

Dr Barry Richardson, *ex-government scientist*

Biolab, *medical referral laboratory, London*

These five highly qualified doctors and the ex-government scientific advisor Barry Richardson all diagnosed chemical injuries, while Biolab, London, used lymphocyte tests to show definite allergy/sensitivity to various pesticides, especially formaldehyde and dimethyl phthalate, which are found in many products, predominantly in the paper industry.

The references at the back of this book prove my point. They show how right Rachel Carson was when she wrote the bestseller *Silent Spring* in 1962. Today the book plays a pivotal role for people who want a cleaner, greener, safer, healthier world in which to live and bring up children, and anyone who wants to be educated in the everyday, insidious, cumulative, synergistic dangers of chemicals and the neurotoxic illnesses they can cause.

There is help out there if you know where to look and if you ask the right people.

CHAPTER 1

Loneliness is the greatest poverty – Mother
Teresa

I was born in 1950 in a maternity hospital in Radcliffe, Manchester, to working class parents. My dad John was on the railways, worked for a time in a cinema and also worked for many years in a nearby paper mill, which would prove to be significant in my later life. My mum Jean worked various jobs, but mostly stayed at home to look after me, my brother Stuart and sister Verna.

I vividly remember my first day at school because I screamed the place down. I'm sure there are plenty of others who are unable to forget that day. Of course, a lot of children cry when first separated from their parents, but I remember not only feeling abandoned but also having a strong feeling of alienation.

One day I was sitting at a round table with my classmates and thinking, *I don't know what I'm doing here.* I just felt odd and out of place. Later in life another ME sufferer once asked me, 'Do you feel like you're a misfit?' She felt the same way that I had felt since childhood. Most people with ME do. If their brain isn't working properly, other people think they are odd.

After a couple of years at school the feelings of alienation subsided but I still never really understood what I wanted to learn. I needed a bigger reason to get up in the morning each day and trudge to school to learn my ABCs. It all seemed so pointless. Consequently I drifted away from academic subjects and my whole world soon revolved around sport. I was a regular in the football first XI at primary school during the year we won both the local league and the cup. I was top goalscorer that season. At secondary school I carried on with the football and added cricket to my sporting talents, winning the cricket cup twice as I became the leading wicket-taker in the cricket first XI. My heroes became cricketers Fred Trueman and Brian Statham, and Denis Law, George Best and Bobby Charlton in football. So, looking back, sport became an outlet for all the anxieties I may have had.

Once I reached the age of fourteen I knew something was wrong. I was playing a match and I realised my coordination on the ball had completely deserted me. From being the top goalscorer, I was now playing like a novice. At first

I brushed it off as just an off day; everybody has an off game once in a while. But I experienced the same in the next match. The situation didn't improve and I got dropped from the team, which devastated me. This was my one passion, the only thing I loved and it was being taken away from me. *If I can't play sport what am I going to do?,* I thought.

Looking back, it is clear to me now that my teenage years, with my body raging with hormones, were the start of my difficulties. Twelve months later I left school and started to feel anxious about the future, a common fear for school leavers: What are you going to do with your life? How will you cope? How will you become a success? I always had a tendency to shyness—I wouldn't speak unless spoken to—which continued through my teens. Because of my condition I did not pass any exams. To use the vernacular of the time, I thought I must be thick. People applied the label to me, and I accepted it.

Much later in life, after I was pensioned from work and the union put a legal team in place to try to gain some compensation, I was put through three-and-a-half hours of psychological testing by neuropsychologist Helen Card. She wrote a fifteen-page report on the tests which ended by stating that I had right-hand side brain damage, and that only 1% of the population would get the results I scored; i.e. those with brain damage.

Martin J Walker mentions a similar case in his 2003 book, *Skewed*, of a boy whose blood sample confirmed a significant increase in autoantibodies against neuronal and glial proteins in his serum. This was also consistent with brain damage from exposure to neurotoxic chemicals such as organophosphate insecticides. I was not alone.

My general IQ score was 118 but my performance level was only 88. On one hand it was shattering to read that report but on the other it certainly explained some things. So technically I *was* a misfit all those years ago as a child when I felt like an outsider—my brain wasn't working like everyone's else. In a village of 500, if 499 are idiots, guess who is classed as the odd one out?

But back in my teens I kept these anxieties to myself, believing I must be thicker and shyer than the average teen. Other times I would be a bit more outgoing but in the main I remained standoffish, which confirmed my lack of confidence.

I have since learned that if the body's cortisol— the flight-or-fight hormone—is low, it can devastate one's confidence. Well, that was me all over. And still is. Following sufficient rest, my life returns to some kind of balance, especially when the weather is warmer. But the body is not running on energy, but rather adrenalin. Eventually the adrenals plummet and I feel washed out. Adrenal burnout is common with

ME–CFS sufferers. The theory is that the adrenal glands are unable to keep pace with the demands of perpetual fight-or-flight arousal.

A lot of medics insist ME symptoms originate in something psychiatric, but equally if you are struggling to maintain a semblance of a normal existence while all this is going on you are going to suffer some psychological lows.

I left school aged fifteen and took a series of general warehouse jobs. Then, aged eighteen, I took a job at Ellison Valdis motor factors, which stored motor manufacturer paints and primers. The firm dealt with potentially hazardous materials, but all the tins and packaging materials were sealed so I had no exposure to anything that could be regarded as detrimental to my health. I got quite friendly with the general manager, who was in his sixties. He was looking forward to retirement while I was on the first rung of the ladder. He discussed his future plans with me and began coaxing me to take over his job. The pay was quite a lot of money at the time and it was a big responsibility ordering paints and supplies to keep the whole operation going. At first I was terrified, but soon the thought of his putting so much trust in me gave me a terrific confidence boost. Maybe I was not so thick after all. *If he thinks I am able to take over on his retirement, I must be good enough,* I thought.

He retired and I got the job. I was happy for a couple of years, the job suited me and the extra money was very welcome. Unfortunately all good things come to an end and so it was with Ellison Valdis. In their wisdom the firm decided to move location and I was not interested in moving with them.

During this time my physical health was good until I was around twenty-three when I had a period of unemployment. Then in September 1974 I got a job with Bury Council as storekeeper, responsible for ordering and stocking all the parts needed for the repairs of council vehicles. They needed an extra storekeeper in what was known as the Dano reclamation plant in Radcliffe, which was run by Greater Manchester Council. The depot collected waste products and rubbish from which they made fertiliser.

There was also an MOT centre for all the council vehicles. I remember thinking nothing of it at the time, but a couple of times a week a powerfully pungent odour emanated from the reclamation plant. I didn't know what they were adding to the reclaimed rubbish to create fertiliser but whatever it was I suspected it was toxic. There was little concern at that time about the long-term effects of fertilisers; nowadays they are regarded in the same light as pesticides.

Around this time I was becoming friendly with a pen friend called Eileen Crook who lived in Mellor in Lancashire, less than an hour away. I had been writing to her since the early 1980s and one day we decided to meet up, which we did, in August 1983. Seven months later she moved in with me. Eileen had an eleven-year-old son (having a child in the house was a new experience to me), but there was an irrepressible chemistry between us so the union worked well.

Six months after she moved in, I called her from work one day (the date, 7 November 1984, is burned into me). She said that when she woke up that morning her right-hand side was completely numb.

'Have you phoned the doctor?' I asked, in a panic.

'Don't bother the doctor.'

Despite Eileen's protestations, I called him and he came that evening. He then sent a consultant who did various tests.

When he returned from the bedroom, I asked, 'Is it MS?'

He said, 'Are you a medic of some kind?'

'No.'

'Then why did you suggest that?'

'I don't know, it just came into my head.'

He said, 'I suspect it *is* multiple sclerosis, but she will have to go to hospital to do more tests.'

Which they did, including a painful lumbar puncture. A couple of days later they confirmed that she had demyelination, a condition that occurs when the protective coating of nerve cells experiences damage. Neurological problems, such as MS, can follow. (See *Stop the 21st Century Killing You* by Dr Paula Baillie-Hamilton, which makes the link between MS and chemical exposures.) After a course of steroids, amongst other drugs, she regained the use of most of her right side. It should go without saying that she was depressed to be off work at the young age of thirty-two with a diagnosis for a serious illness.

In 1983 the powers that be decided to close the garage at Radcliffe. I thought I would lose my job, but fortunately I got a phone call telling me there was an opportunity in the parks/grounds department, which I jumped at. I was only thirty-three and thought it would be brilliant working outside during the summer months. In fact, Alfred, my mum's dad, had finished his working life as a groundsman, so it seemed fitting that I should follow in his footsteps.

Initially I was part of a three-man team working out of a Land Rover pulling a trailer with all the gear responsible for the upkeep of the local school playing fields, gardens and sports pitches. We marked them out for summer sports in the spring (athletics tracks, etc) and winter sports in the autumn (football pitches). I loved it.

One day at work in 1984 after using a dry, granular-type weedkiller, I returned to the Land Rover and suddenly felt tense and anxious and my mouth went completely dry. It made me worried because nothing unusual had happened that day. I took a breather and it soon passed off. Neither of my work colleagues said they felt anything untoward, so I kept my symptoms to myself. But, looking back, my reaction indicated, for the first time, that there was something toxic in the weedkiller.

The chemical in the weedkiller has since been taken off the market; in fact two of the three pesticide brand names are no longer on sale. One, Casoron-G, had an active ingredient called dichlobenil, which is an organic compound generally used for weed control in amenity, non-crop areas and aquatic situations. It remained for sale until March 2009.

Anyway, I put my reaction down to just 'one of those things'. I didn't make the link to the pesticides we used because at the time one would have assumed—I certainly did anyway—that something publicly available would have passed all health and safety laws, so why would it affect me?

In the summer of 1985, Chris the foreman said it was time to mark out the athletics tracks on all the school playing fields. We had always made the initial markings with creosote, which burned in the lines on the grass before we used Rainstay white line paint, after which we would freshen up the lines once a week. When it came to using the creosote that year we were told that it had been banned for use at school because a child had fallen on the grass and received a minor burn from the chemical. Consequently everyone was scratching their heads, wondering what we were going to use to burn in the lines. Then Chris came out of the office carrying two large containers of Roundup, a herbicide, at that time produced by Monsanto. He suggested we put a small solution into the paint so we could do the two jobs at once. We all thought that was a great idea because it saved us time and got the job done quicker. The system worked well and, at the time, I had no apparent side effects from using it.

Much later, after I was pensioned off from work, I got a report from ex-government scientist Barry Richardson which suggested there may have been a chemical reaction triggered by mixing the two solutions. Richardson noted that Rainstay was not on the register of biocides and that the reaction could have created a phosphine gas, a colourless, flammable, very toxic gas compound. He also suggested that an organophosphate could have been created by mixing it into the galvanised steel marking machine itself.

Once again, even though there was a fishy, pungent odour emanating from the Rainstay mixture, we didn't question it because we assumed the solutions were safe. Although we only used this new solution for about three weeks, i.e., the length of time it took us to mark out all the school grounds, once they were burned in we would regularly retrace the lines with the lining paint.

In 1986 I left the Prestwich three-man team to move to Whitefield to a former girls' grammar school, now known as Philips High School, where my grandfather used to work. They had a resident groundsman at the school who was leaving. I replaced him. I remained there until I finished working in 1992.

When it came to the winter and summer changeovers on the playing fields I used the same system shown me by my foreman, and because I was the only person working there, at the end of the day I would often be left with a residue in the bottom of the marking machine. I couldn't pour it down the drain, so I was unsure what to do with the leftovers. My priority was to keep it away from the children, so I secured it in the locked shed, believing that was the safest course of action. The only person who entered the hut was me—up to three or four times a day to get tools or machines —when I would have breathed in what had been brewing overnight. The toxic OPs were waiting for me every morning I opened up the store for work.

I would arrive at work each day and like clockwork I would experience a runny nose. In November 1989 the GP diagnosed vasomotor rhinitis. "Vaso" means blood vessels and "motor" refers to the nerves, which innervates nasal tissue and the blood vessels. The doctor prescribed baclofen and an inhaler twice at night. A mild treatment to most people, but to me it felt like some kind of drug trip.

Day by day I felt more seriously unwell. But my initial symptoms were not only physical; I was also undergoing an emotional rollercoaster which could be seen in my unexplained irritability. I got up one morning and was so wound up in a fit of temper for no reason I smashed the telephone into a glass table.

To get to the school, about a mile and a half away, I had to pass Stand golf course. As I walked on that stretch my stomach started churning and I was overcome with a feeling of dread. Later I was convinced that the course had been using chemical spraying to keep the weeds at bay, which added to the already high level of toxicity in my system. Around this time I was also bitten by an insect on my wrist at work, which drew blood, for which I had a tetanus jab.

By October 1988 I experienced what all the medics will tell you are the initial symptoms of ME: a persistent flu-like illness and severe fatigue. I was off work for two weeks, which was very unusual for me. I was whacked, as if all my energy was spent, and my body was shaking like an internal shiver.

I returned to work after a fortnight even though I felt only 40% back to normal. I was scared to lose my job, but I was equally scared that I may have been physically unable to *do* the job. I soldiered on but over the next few months I had to take regular short spells off work to recuperate. I would force myself to continue but eventually my body couldn't take it anymore and it would crash. No one knew what was wrong with me, including my GP.

I struggled on at work until 1991. On 25 April I was doing the summer changeover with a groundsman from another school and mixing the chemicals as I had always done. At about 3 p.m. I was pouring the herbicide into the white lining agent when all of a sudden my face started tingling, then my arms. Then I went dizzy. I had to sit down. The guy with me asked if I was okay. I told him how I felt and said I couldn't continue the job. He could see the seriousness of the situation and was good enough to run me home. Eileen was in bed with a bad back so I didn't want to disturb her. I stayed in the lounge and bent over to take off my shoes. When I stood up the room started going round in the most severe case of vertigo I have ever experienced. I felt drained and unusually cold. My breathing was shallow and I felt excruciating itching. I went upstairs to have a wash and try to bring myself around. I looked in the mirror and was horrified at what I saw. My clammy face was white as a ghost.

I made my way back downstairs. Within a few minutes my breathing became more and more laboured. It crossed my mind to call 999, but the sheer effort to get up and reach for the phone was too much for me. I knew that if I had tried to stand up and make the call I would have made a bad situation worse. I sat back in the chair and forced myself to regulate my breathing, which was becoming more desperate by the minute. I was at crisis point and could not fathom what was happening to me.

By this time I had convinced myself that my time was up and that I was about to fade away. I simply lay back and waited for the worst. After forty minutes I came to and could feel my breathing get a bit easier. Eventually I returned to some kind of normality. With my mind at ease, I either blacked out or fell asleep. An hour later I woke up feeling terrible, so I went to bed and spent the night in fits and starts of sleep. Next morning I felt like I had the hangover from hell, as if I had been on a three-day alcohol binge. Then I was overtaken with nausea.

I tried to think logically about the course of events that day and reached the conclusion that the cause must have been the chemicals at work. I called in sick the next day and explained what I thought may have been the cause. The foreman brought me some forms intended to log the incident as a work accident, although he didn't seem too happy about. It later dawned on me that he may have been part of the problem because he had brought two 5-gallon drums of the white lining agent plus an unlabelled herbicide, marked in red felt tip pen "Poison".

Whatever his involvement or culpability in the accident, at least I was satisfied that it had been documented. I took two weeks off work. My employer, Bury Council, sent a doctor from the Employment Medical Advisory Service who listened to my story. A few weeks later a report was sent which stressed the itching but seemed to skirt around the possible cause and most severe symptoms in an attempt to pacify everyone. But the itching was the least of the symptoms. What about the fact that I could hardly breathe and the terrible hangover immediately afterwards?

Five years later, in June 1996, I got my GP to refer me to a Dr Davies in Taunton who had been seeing farmers who had been complaining of similarly debilitating symptoms following sheep dipping. (Professor Behan had just published his research paper on ME victims and sheep dippers suffering from a flu-like illness, severe fatigue, anxiety/depression, low concentration, bowel problems, etc., all symptoms that are listed in the Health and Safety Executive [HSE] document.)

MS17 poisoning by organophosphates fits exactly with sheep dippers using OP sheep dips, and of course people like myself working in horticulture. But where was OP exposure coming from with lots of other ME victims? When Dr Davies's report stated that I had a cholinergic crisis (relating to the nerves) from chemicals at work.

I don't usually go in for conspiracy theories but I began to think there may have been some kind of cover-up.

I returned to work but was kept away from marking out the fields, so managed to avoid all the (by now suspect) chemicals. I lasted until the end of 1991. On 4 January 1992 I suddenly felt unwell at work with all the old symptoms and had to go home. I would never return to work. I was forty-one.

CHAPTER 2

'Doctor, doctor, they've poisoned my brain.'
'Nay, nay, nay, patient, please refrain.'
'But doctor, doctor, you're being so unkind.'
'No, my patient, it's all in your mind.'

For six months I was in limbo. The GP continued to sign my rolling sick note from January to June of 1992 before I received a letter from work explaining that as it looked likely I would not return to work, would I consider accepting a pension. Even though they accepted no responsibility for my exposure to the dangerous chemicals, Bury Council accepted that I was sick enough to be pensioned off. This was not always a given because many council staff were suspected of what they called 'working the ticket', which meant getting early retirement on health grounds and immediately starting another job. It seems to me now that my employers were taking the cautious line to let me go with an acceptable pension and hoping the problem didn't come back to haunt them in the future. There was no way I could have faced another job in the condition I was in.

Even though I was now away from the organophosphates at work, my energy level continued to diminish week by week. I went to the GP who had always been helpful and sympathetic to the situation (not that he ever acknowledged that I had been poisoned by chemicals at work). He suggested that some of my symptoms might be in the mind. He would not be the last medic to suggest the symptoms were psychosomatic. I would later discover that he must have been aware of at least the possibility of chemical poisoning because every GP in the UK had been sent—in that very month—a warning of the prevalence of pesticide incidents at work.

Despite my relative youth, I agreed to accept the pension. If I couldn't work, what other option did I have? To jump through the administrative hoops for my employer, I was sent to another couple of doctors to confirm my inability to work, which approved my pension on health grounds. I still don't know what was written in the report, but I do know that they liaised with my GP to agree a form of words to cover my disability. From that point on, my GP always wrote on my sick notes "Pesticide toxicity", which may have been prompted by the conversation with the other doctors. Who knows?

I had been with the council eighteen years all told, and they made up my time with another six years pension contributions, plus I had an ongoing sick payment, which was probably the best I could have hoped for. These two payments may seem generous but they did not amount to what I was earning in the job. A worrying concern at the time was the fact that Eileen and I had just moved house and taken on a larger mortgage. Talk about bad timing. Unfortunately the new location was very rural and the house backed onto a farm which was the worst move we could have made, plus there was a golf course not far away, which presented the potential danger of chemical spraying. We managed to move to my present house in 2002.

Shortly after leaving work I got a call from someone at my union, NUPE (National Union of Public Employees), who asked for an update on my situation. She asked if I wanted to make a claim for compensation. I had not considered the possibility of such action but now that I had the mortgage around my neck, and if in fact they *had* done me harm, I agreed.

'Right,' she said, 'I shall put the claim in motion.'

Shortly afterwards I got a letter that asked me to visit one of their solicitors in Manchester, who suggested we get two or three independent opinions on my condition. The first one was

Professor Blaine, the director of the Medical Toxicology Centre at Newcastle University, who seemed eminently qualified to offer an opinion on my case.

One snowy day in February 1994 Eileen and I went off to Newcastle. Dr Blaine listened to my story and made copious notes as he considered what had happened to me. He wrote a report which didn't say anything concrete, and basically sat on the fence. Of course I had told him about the mixing of the Rainstay but the report only mentioned the herbicide, not the mixing of the chemicals.

Alarm bells started going off inside me. In fact his report said little more than what the health & safety sheets stated about the herbicide (which of course were, and still are, written by the manufacturer—in this case, Monsanto). But Dr Blaine did say that many COSHH regulations were routinely broken, and claims have recently been won in the USA.

In 2018 I read about a former school groundsman called Dewayne Johnson who won £226 million in a court settlement after jurors found against Monsanto, which owned Roundup until the firm was bought by German pharmaceutical group Bayer. The professional grade version (Roundup Ranger Pro) contributed substantially to Mr Johnson's terminal cancer, the jury said. Emma Hockridge, head of policy at the

Soil Association, said the ruling was a dramatic blow to the pesticide industry, and told a British newspaper, 'This is a landmark case which highlights not only the problems caused by glyphosate [the active ingredient in Roundup] but also the whole system of pesticide use.'

After eight weeks of proceedings the jury found Monsanto acted with malice, oppression or fraud, and should be punished for its conduct.

Robert F Kennedy Junior, son of the late US senator and nephew of former President John F Kennedy, said, 'The jury sent a message to the Monsanto boardroom that they have to change the way they do business. You not only see many people injured, you see the corruption of public officials, the capture of agencies that are supposed to protect us from pollution, and the falsification of science.'

In 2015 the World Health Organisation rated glyphosate as a group 2A carcinogen, which ranks it as "a substance that probably causes cancer in people". In 2017, the state of California added glyphosate to its Proposition 65 list, which requires Roundup to carry a warning label if sold in Califiornia. Monsanto now faces nearly 5,000 other lawsuits across the US.

Against this trend, the EU voted to renew a five-year licence of glyphosate in November 2017, despite the cancer fears. The UK was one of eighteen countries that voted for the contract, even though France planned to ban using glyphosate within three years. I also wondered why the HSE didn't investigate synergistic effects from mixing chemicals.

Dr Blaine suggested that I was suffering from PTSD as a consequence of a temporal association with the industrial accident in April 1991. It was like a kick in the teeth. In effect he was suggesting there might be a psychological cause, but side-stepped the physical one. However, in legal terms the PTSD diagnosis was still claimable. The best that could be said for the consultation was that at least he didn't close any doors in terms of bringing a claim for compensation.

The unions did nothing about the report except to send me to another doctor at the National Poisons Unit at Guy's Hospital in London. I was greatly encouraged by this appointment. Where better to go?

Eileen and I took the train and spent an overnight in London in preparation for the next morning's appointment with who I believed were the top people in the country. I faced a panel of four physicians who listened to all the details—I was by now an expert in the retelling of my tale. Occasionally the team leader asked a question pertaining to my level of stress.

At one point he asked, 'I believe your partner has multiple sclerosis.'

I said, 'Yes, she was diagnosed in 1984.'

'How did you feel about that?'

I knew exactly what he was getting at: *Partner is ill, I had to do lots of running around, plus I had a job of work... perhaps it all got too much for me.* I was sure that was the line he was taking.

I just said, 'Whoa! I'm a very forthright person and I like to be honest at all times and I speak my mind. I know what you're suggesting and it's out of order.'

He sat back in his chair as if trying to weigh me up. He didn't like being challenged.

I continued, 'I'm not having it, laying the blame for my condition on anxiety. Once these chemicals have been investigated scientifically and shown in black and white that there is no impact on my health then I will accept that maybe I am just getting myself worked up. But until that date, no!'

I wondered if he had read Dr Richard Mackarness's books *Not All in the Mind* and *Chemical Victims*.

They got me to perform a number of tests, after which I was ready to leave. He came to me holding a big folder.

'I want you to take these documents with you and fill in the questionnaire,' he said, 'then please send them back.'

I took the folder and didn't think much more about it. By this time I was happy just to get out of the place. On the train home I opened the folder which revealed a series of about fifty questions pertaining to my psychiatric state. None of the questions asked about the chemicals. Some were extremely intrusive, two of which stood out: "Do you believe in Martians?" and "Have you ever sexually assaulted anyone?"

I looked at Eileen and said, 'What on earth is this nonsense?'

I got home and phoned someone I had become friendly with due to our mutual suffering. Annette Griffiths was from the Pesticide Exposure Group of Sufferers (PEGS) who had worked in a care home and suffered the same condition as me. The home had been sprayed regularly by a pest control company who were all suited and booted in protective gear but the staff and residents had to inhale it all unprotected.

Anyway, I told her I had just returned from Guy's, a trauma she had experienced some time before. She was appalled and wanted to compare notes about the daft questionnaire we were given.

Then her tone changed and she got a little more excited.

'I've got some news for you,' she said.

'What's that?'

'*Panorama* has been on to me about making a documentary about OPs. They're looking to feature someone who does not work in the care sector or on a farm.'

When Annette referred to farm workers she raised a subject with which I had recently become familiar: the plight of Britain's sheep dippers.

In 1951 a government working group produced a report for the Ministry of Agriculture, Fisheries and Food (MAFF) on toxic chemicals in agriculture, which identified the risks of agricultural organophosphate pesticides and recommended that they be labelled as "deadly poison". Nevertheless, from 1976 to 1992 MAFF made sheep-dipping compulsory—while simultaneously insisting the OP containers be labelled as potentially hazardous.

In the early 1980s the Health and Safety Executive guidance sheet MS17 was produced, called "Biological Monitoring of Workers Exposed to OP Pesticides", which spelled out the dangers... OP pesticides *could penetrate protective clothing* and that *repeated exposure may have had irreversible cumulative neurological effects.* Incredibly, it was never circulated to farmers, GPs, vets or hospital doctors. Also, it mentioned that one of the early signs of exposure to pesticides can be vasomotor rhinitis, for which I had been treated back in 1989.

This was a time bomb waiting to go off. In the 1980s and 1990s hundreds of farm workers and their families reported symptoms including fatigue, memory loss, weakness, joint and muscle pain and depression, which they suspected was due to exposure to the OPs in sheep dip. The government denied that there was a clear link, while at the same time, in 1992, decreeing that sheep dipping would no longer be compulsory.

The deliberate suppression of the MS17 document undoubtedly exacerbated, if not caused, much of the suffering experienced by farmers, who had no idea what was wrong with them. What was worse was being confronted by the ignorance of health professionals.

The day after Annette's call about the BBC documentary I was contacted by a researcher called Faisal Ali who explained what they wanted to do. In preparation for the filming he arranged a meeting with Annette together with another nurse and me in Chester. We had lunch and we told him the story. It all looked very promising; finally we would be able to bring these problems to light. What better way to do it than on BBC's flagship current affairs programme?

Off he went. A week went by. Curious to know how the documentary was progressing, I phoned Annette.

'Have you heard from Faisal Ali?'

'Nothing.'

That was the last we heard from *Panorama*. Could it be that someone *up there* had pulled the plug on this controversial subject?

Back to 1994 and the doctor consultations. After the union received the reports from

Newcastle and Guy's someone from the union called me.

'Sorry, Brian,' she said, 'we have done two investigations and don't find any grounds to carry on with the case.'

I was naturally disappointed but at least we had made a serious attempt at getting a scientific explanation for my illness. I now just had to get on with life the best I could.

CHAPTER 3

Starve the ego, feed the soul

In 1992, after moving into our new house, I started redecorating, which included some painting. Afterwards I felt terrible. That night I felt as if I was suffering a toxic hangover. I tried to brush it off and returned to the painting the following day, but it got no better. I was convinced that the paint was the cause of my ailment.

I saw my GP who made an appointment at Manchester Royal Infirmary (MRI) where, believing I had an allergic reaction, they did the skin prick test to measure the presence of IgE antibodies. I went back a week later for the results, which suggested I was not allergic because my score was only 34 on the scale and needed to be over 100 to be allergic. I was bemused.

I went back a couple more times for more tests, but then they sent a letter to my GP saying that I was suffering from depression. I was astounded and wondered how they could equate the two. It just didn't make sense to me. Their response seemed to me to be an easy answer: if they can't find a cause they call you depressed and stressed or say you have a virus. The last doctor I saw at MRI said that he was soon leaving for Australia and that if I ever discovered the cause of my condition would I contact him. He gave me his number. To give him his due he really wanted to know what was wrong with me. I did some more digging and discovered that the IgE allergy test was only one option for detecting allergies, there were others which could have been more appropriate. I mentioned it to the GP but he didn't think it was worth pursuing.

My reaction to the paint made me realise that I was becoming hypersensitive to all sorts of chemicals and toxins, which I now planned to avoid at all costs. I searched my house for anything that could potentially harm me. I didn't realise the cocktail of toxins I had stored under my sink, which all had to be thrown away.

To this day you will not find a chemical or cleaning product in my bungalow. I use lemon juice and bicarbonate of soda to clean the bulk of the house, and cider vinegar for the bathroom. There are some eco friendly washing-up liquids with which I wash the dishes and use in the washing machine. I can't go near bleach. The last time I used it I was on the bed for days. I am so hypersensitive now, which is why I became so receptive to reiki, which I shall come to shortly.

Later I saw a report in the paper from someone who was an agronomist—an expert in the science of soil management and crop production—who spent much of her time rooting around in farmer's hay lofts. Of course, all the hay had been sprayed with God knows what. Eventually she got what I had (and still have)—chemical sensitivity syndrome. She ended up having to move to Cornwall to live in a caravan. I saved the cutting and sent it to the head of MRI immunology. To my surprise, a fortnight later he replied to say that the increased sensitivity from organophosphorus poisoning had a biochemical basis not an immunological one, so sadly he was unable to help me in his clinic.

Sometimes I felt like a lone voice in the OP wilderness, especially after meeting doctors and specialists who took the first opportunity to lay the blame for all my ailments on my psychological make-up: anxiety, stress, psychosomatic conditions and all the rest. I knew there were other sufferers out there—more than the few I had met at support groups—but the subject of OP poisoning had not yet filtered down to the general public. That required the media to take it seriously.

In 1994, campaigning *Sunday Telegraph* journalist Christopher Booker began writing about the effects of OPs on sheep dippers. It was a cause he felt passionately about. When he got his teeth into something he wouldn't let go. During decades in journalism he banged the drum for many causes: from the scepticism of climate change to the evils of the EU, from British social history to modernist architecture. He was even a founder of the satirical magazine *Private Eye*.

He took up the cause of farm workers who, following the 1976 government regulation, were compelled to dip their sheep in a chemical compound to eliminate two nasty parasites, scab and blowfly, which eat into the animals' fleeces. The only safety warning on the chemical used was "Handle with Care", so the farmers supposed that they were generally safe to use. The chemical solution contained organophosphates. Some years later many farmers started coming down with mystery illnesses such as muscle twitching, dizziness, exhaustion and loss of memory. Some doctors diagnosed ME — myalgic encephalomyelitis.

Chris Booker wrote about the link between OPs and ME–CFS after a fellow journalist called Maureen Cleave was overcome by dizziness and later suffered tiredness, depression, memory impairment, aching muscles and headaches, and eventually had to retire with ME. The link between

ME–CFS and exposure to organophosphorus chemicals had already been investigated by Professor Peter Behan of Glasgow University. He noted that victims suffered from severe impairment of their immune system, and in 1996 produced a research document entitled *CFS: A delayed reaction to chronic low dose organophosphate exposure.*

Professor Behan noted that abnormal results in the OP users' group were the same found in ME–CFS patients given the same tests, and that the symptoms of chronic organophosphate poisoning were identical to those of ME–CFS.

Armed with that report, Chris Booker now considered how so many people had come to be exposed to these "neurotoxic chemicals". He discovered that lactating cows were treated with OPs, so perhaps they could enter our milk; vegetables were sprayed with OPs; and grain was treated with OPs (intended to protect it in storage) so perhaps it could persist in flour for bread. Although the quantities entering the body may be minute, OPs work cumulatively, gradually eroding the nervous system and the body's immunity. Subsequent exposure to small amounts of OPs in everyday life could be shown to trigger a serious reaction in patients. It was by now becoming increasingly difficult to avoid its use as a fire retardant in home products.

Booker's investigations widened to include other compounds and solutions that contained OPs, which he included in an illuminating article published in the Reader's Digest under the headline "Poisoned by Order–Plight of our Sheep Farmers". He quoted me in the article as someone who was forced to retire after suffering a workplace injury. He wrote:

"In June 1992 the Government announced, with no clear explanation, that compulsory sheep dipping would end. At least any future damage would be limited. Official spokesmen repeatedly insisted that there was 'no scientific evidence' to link sick farmers with OPs. There was therefore no reason for banning their use. [It is clear to me that this was an attempt by the Government to distance itself from any future claims.]

But there was *clinical* evidence. That October, the National Poisons Unit advised on a small study of farmers that there was a 'medical problem from occupational exposure'. The following year the NPU confirmed it had 'identified patients with chronic health effects associated with exposure to sheep dip'. It concluded, 'Their condition is a matter for concern.'

More and more victims were coming forward, many of whom had no connection with sheep dipping. Brian Hopkinson was a council groundsman in Bury, Greater Manchester. In 1985 the use of creosote to mark out playing fields was banned, so his employers gave him an OP-based herbicide to use instead. Over the next few years he suffered from a permanent flu-like illness. 'Then, in 1991, I had a violent reaction while using chemicals. My health got so bad that I was forced to give up work.'"

Chris Booker had contacted me through another campaigner, Elizabeth Sigmund, who ran a support group for sheep dip sufferers. She spent many years as an environmental activist, campaigning against research into and production of chemical and biological weapons, nerve agents, and the use of organophosphates in sheep dip. The nerve agents in chemical and biological weapons were closely related to the OP pesticides in sheep dip. In fact, the Health and Safety Executive had published a paper that contained crucial information about the dangers of OP sheep dip.

This was all good news as far as ME–CFS sufferers were concerned. These articles were starting to create doubt in people's minds about the wisdom of using OPs.

Following Booker's 1994 article in the *Telegraph,* the news and current affairs programme *BBC Northwest* contacted me. In

April 1996 I got a call from the journalist Martin Henfield who said they were doing a piece on the dangers of toxins hiding in people's sheds, etc. He had been given my number from one of the self-help groups. 'By all means,' I said.

The following day a journalist showed up with a cameraman and I told them what had happened to me. The piece also included an interview with a professor of bio-chemistry from Liverpool University. The interview, in which the professor explained how everyday toxins can have a debilitating effect on people's lives, was aired a few days later, and included a short interview with me.

A couple of days after the broadcast I received a phone call from a Liverpool groundsman who said that he was suffering from the same condition as me after being asked to use similar chemicals at work. I believe he was also pensioned off.

A fortnight later I got another phone call from a researcher on the Radio 4 programme *Farming Today*. She came to the house for the interview which was aired shortly after.

It mattered little to me personally to be featured in the media in this way but I was glad that the issue was being discussed, not only for other sufferers but for the wider population. It was finally being taken seriously.

Eighteen months later Christopher Booker wrote a piece under the headline "Why the OP story cannot be told", which suggested the full story would be too explosive for the government. I believed then that the powers that be were putting pressure on the media to drop the story. Chris never wrote about it again—the information has stopped being disseminated, allowing the disease to flourish.

In 1989, while dipping her sheep through a tank of organophosphorus chemicals, the Countess of Mar got a splash of chemicals on her foot. Three weeks later she developed headaches and muscular pains. She was subsequently diagnosed with chronic fatigue syndrome. Since then she has campaigned for better support for CFS sufferers and better regulation of OPs and founded *Forward-ME* to co-ordinate the activities of a broad spectrum of organisations working with ME–CFS patients.

Lady Mar told a Liverpudlian friend of mine and fellow sufferer, John, that the full story of the dangers of OPs could not be told because it would bankrupt the country. John replied that if the story is *not* told, the country would be bankrupt anyway because no one would be able to work.

Some scientists are now widening their investigations into organophosphates away from farming and industrial chemicals to seemingly benign everyday activities. Scientists and doctors from the US, France and Australia have identified what they call aerotoxic syndrome, which they claim is caused by exposure to toxic oil fumes present on most commercial jets. They say that passengers breathe 'bleed air' drawn unfiltered from the compression section of the engines into the cabin. Oil leaks in the engine seals can release a potent mix of potentially toxic fumes containing OPs. That 'smelly socks' odour you can smell on aircraft? That could be toxic, they say. The hidden illness is known to affect the central nervous system and brain, causing a range of acute symptoms and long-term ill health. Passengers and crew disembark aeroplanes thinking they've got the flu but are actually suffering from aerotoxic syndrome. Remember, ME–CFS also starts with flu-like symptoms. Of course, the airline industry plays down the risks but, while aerotoxic syndrome remains largely unrecognised, thousands of people continue to suffer every day without knowing about this hidden health and safety hazard.

This brings me to one of my central contentions in my illness. It is so difficult for the medical profession to pin down the cause of ME–CFS symptoms because they need to see a direct cause and effect. But this does not take into account the synergistic, cumulative effect of exposure to otherwise benign chemicals in everyday life.

So, to be fair to my ex-employers, it was not just the exposure to their chemicals that brought on my condition; it was also the cumulative effect of chemicals in the environment.

And I can go back even further. I believe my genes were damaged while my mother was carrying me in the womb. The chemical firm Theodore St Just was situated 100 metres from her home in Whitefield. I would spend a lot of time there in my early years. I do remember foul, strange smells when visiting. Also the local press were reporting lots of residents complaining to the council of obnoxious smells emanating from the chemical plant. The complaints became so vociferous that the council agreed to a rate reduction to compensate. If only it were that simple. The real point surely is what was I and everyone else in the vicinity being exposed to? I recently learned that an explosion took place at this plant in 1957, when I was aged seven. One poor man was blown through the roof, another lost the sight in one eye.

CHAPTER 4

Pointing the Way

In 1995 the campaigner Elizabeth Sigmund called and told me to buy a copy of the *Guardian* the following day. Apparently there was going to be an article in the magazine section by Barry Richardson about how he had been helping the New Zealand Government with their investigations into Sudden Infant Death Syndrome (SIDS). He had recommended they withdraw the sale of waterproof mattresses that had been treated with certain chemicals. He discovered that when a child's urine came into contact with the mattress a tiny amount of phospine gas was being formed, which could potentially be fatal to an infant, especially if lying face down.

It put me in mind of the time I had great difficulty breathing and had to leave work after mixing the Rainstay with the mystery chemical. I wrote to Barry Richardson, explaining my situation, and asked if he believed I could have suffered/was suffering from a similar effect. He replied and said that, yes, I could have been affected by either a reaction of the two chemicals or a reaction between one of the chemicals and the galvanised marking machine itself. It was a theory I had not yet considered.

I believed he was the man to help me make my case, but then he was such an eminent scientist, what kind of fee would he charge to investigate my case? He was interested enough to ask for the name of the solicitor acting for me. I had to tell him, 'No one!'

I eventually found a firm of Manchester solicitors who agreed to pursue the case on my behalf, but the problem was that it was past the limitation of three years since the accident. Despite this drawback, somehow the lawyers convinced Bury Council to agree to a pre-trial hearing in March 2001 at Oldham County Court: Hopkinson v Bury Council.

It was my big day in court. The council brought a barrister up from London to represent them, so I could see they were taking it seriously. I brought Eileen along for some support. I told my story simply and straightforwardly, I could do no more. Now it was up to the judge. He adjourned the case for a week, while he deliberated. We then returned to the court for his comments. He read out his long judgment, which initially seemed to side with the defendant, but eventually he declared that he would allow my case to go forward on what was called a Section 33 clause, mainly because of the detailed report I had compiled.

As we were leaving, the council solicitor turned to me with a sneer and said that my case would be laughed out of court. My reply to him is unprintable!

A week later the firm of solicitors representing me said they would prefer not to continue the claim solely for OP poisoning, but rather for a cocktail of chemicals, which would give a greater possibility of winning the case. I refused. I smelt a rat, especially when they told me they would be changing the judge. I also learned that there were a lot of sheep dippers with cases pending. If I won in court on OP poisoning it would set a precedent and open the flood gates. More food for thought.

I then found another solicitor to represent me. He sent me to Glasgow Southern General Hospital to see a consultant neurologist for tests. The so-called expert said my condition was probably due to mucus membrane irritation coupled with anxiety and chronic fatigue syndrome, essentially leaving the diagnosis open to possible psychological problems. This was soul destroying.

The doctor must have had a change of heart because two years later I came across an article written by the same consultant in a journal called *Pesticide News* which highlighted the dangers of organophosphates to people exposed to chemicals at work and in their homes. His evidence was being used to support a case against a large chemical company to establish whether children suffered from the effects of OPs.

Meanwhile, quite naturally, the pressure from the stress of the whole affair was building inside me, which led to a series of relapses. I felt terrible: sky-high stress coupled with kitten-like weakness. It was like having a nervous breakdown without end. At any one time I felt as though I was experiencing the lowest of the low. It couldn't possibly get any worse, could it?

Then it *did* get worse.

When I heard that one of my allies, Barry Richardson, was retiring, my life collapsed. I was distraught because I had put in all that work and now had nothing to show for it. I also wondered if Professor Richardson's sudden retirement was linked to a bigger picture. The plot thickened. I was then sent to see a pharmacologist in Birmingham by the opposition solicitors. I was struck by how many times he kept saying that I had *not* been exposed to OPs.

Nevertheless, the case continued. In December 2001 yet another solicitor took on my case, in fact she came to my house with a barrister to get some background details and convince me to carry on. I was exhausted and ready to throw in the towel on the whole affair, but they kept up the pressure.

They even warned me that if I pulled out of the case there was a possibility that Bury Council could sue me for wasting their time with a vexatious claim.

The barrister asked, 'Don't you want to win £100,000 damages?'

I replied, 'I don't want £100 million if it means not telling the truth.'

They both left shaking their heads.

The consequence of that meeting was that my already poor health nosedived. I was bedridden and in a terrible state: sweating, hot and cold fevers, uncontrollable shaking, and tachycardia that sent my stress levels through the roof. I hit rock bottom for four days and four nights with not a wink of sleep and not a bite to eat. One night Eileen called a doctor at 2 a.m. All he could say was that it was a deterioration of my existing OP condition.

Eileen was fraught with worry the whole time. By now I believe I had developed multiple chemical sensitivity (MCS), an admittedly controversial diagnosis attributed to exposure to low levels of commonly used chemicals.

Despite feeling dreadful, somehow I had to get to my GP to take something to calm me down. Just before Christmas 2001 he suggested taking beta blockers that would reduce my blood pressure by blocking the effects of my surging adrenaline which was working overtime. I was always sceptical of taking drugs (and still am) so I agreed to the new medication on condition that I only take a child's dose. We agreed that I would take 5 ml morning and night. After the first dose I felt like someone had plunged me into a deep well of darkness. The surreal feeling lasted half an hour. Once my body got used to the shock, the drug did calm me down a little for a few days. But soon my breathing became laboured and I ended up in Bolton Royal Infirmary.

The doctors in A&E didn't know what to do with me, so I lay there on the trolley wondering what fresh hell I would be put through. At 1 a.m. someone came to my bedside and asked me how I was.

'Who are you?' I asked.

'The hospital psychologist.'

I might have guessed. Later I learned that the A&E report sent to my GP listed "panic attack" as my condition. By this time so many people were trying to tell me I was mad that I wondered myself. But I kept remembering the two books written by Dr Richard Mackerness. By this stage even Eileen thought I had psycho problems and that I was imagining the dangers of chemicals everywhere. The whole situation was driving a wedge between us.

I later obtained information leaflets on the beta blocker. Underneath a skull and crossbones it stated "Do not give to patients with allergies". This was more confirmation that I had suffered an allergic reaction to the beta blocker and not a panic attack, as diagnosed. I began to wonder how many other people get insulted by the medical profession's ignorance of biochemical sensitisation of the autonomic and central nervous system. The whole episode should have been documented as a yellow card incident, which indicates an adverse reaction to the drug.

In July 2002 we moved to the bungalow in which I still live. Moving house is stressful enough if you are in good health but with my condition I was knocked for six. I was on the bed for three months.

CHAPTER 5

If heaven sends you reiki to help you to heal
Be sure to embrace it with zest and with zeal.
Then you may hear an angel whisper on the
breeze
Take care of the healers, they don't grow on trees.
B. Hopkinson

Around this time Eileen happened to come home one evening with a local free paper in which I saw an ad for reiki healing by a practitioner called Barbara Gardiner in nearby Whitefield. I had no idea what reiki was but was intrigued enough to call the number and go along for a couple of sessions. Each treatment took about an hour. I lay on a treatment table fully clothed and Barbara lay her hands on me. It seemed a strange thing to be doing, but considering all that I had gone through I was ready to try anything, however unconventional.

From the first session I felt a glowing radiance flowing through me. After a few more visits I could feel myself relaxing in both mind and body, as if the scales of trauma were falling from my eyes. I rediscovered a sense of wellbeing that had eluded me for years. Finally I had found a method of healing that could reach inside me and somehow make my life bearable again.

The word reiki comes from two Japanese words: *Rei* "God's Wisdom or the Higher Power" and *Ki* "Life force energy". It is spiritual in nature but is not a religion; there is no 'teaching' in the traditional sense. It is based on the idea that an unseen life force energy flows through each and every body. If this life force is low or suppressed, we are more likely to get sick or feel stress; if the life force energy is high, we are more capable of being happy and healthy.

I learned that people used the technique to reduce pain, stress and fatigue, help manage symptoms of existing ailments, reduce side effects of medications (not in my case as I cannot tolerate any), and support recovery from injuries or surgery. It sounded like a wonder cure.

After I was fully convinced of its benefits, Barbara asked if I would like to learn to practice reiki. Yes, please. The level one reiki techniques were transferred to me during what's known as an attunement. This allowed me to use reiki to heal myself when I needed some spiritual intervention. Neuroscientists say that we only use 10% of the brain, and I believed that reiki might help me tap into some of the other 90%. (See the book, *Proof of Heaven* by Dr Eben Alexander.)

About this time I was invited to take part in another BBC interview, this time on Radio 4.

'What is reiki?' asked BBC presenter Winifred Robinson on the lunchtime radio programme *You and Yours*. I told Winifred that it is a life force energy that calms both the nervous system and the troubles of the mind.

'But where does it come from?' she asked.

'From the universe,' I said. 'When we are brought up we are taught only to believe things that we can perceive, but we all accept that electricity exists, and that power is generated by wind without knowing exactly how. In a sense, reiki is just another form of energy, but one that you can feel. Firstly by heat coming from the hands of a practitioner when giving a healing.'

I hope I gave Winifred and her 3 million listeners something to think about. Some people come to reiki hoping it might be a quick fix, but that is definitely not how it works. Many have been what I call 'brainised' by mainstream media, which tells us that if you have any ailments you must either take drugs or cut it out/chop it off. Reiki will help you cope when your problems cannot be cut away.

I can say now that it helped me immensely with my untreatable poisoning. Following my attunements reiki altered the way I thought, felt and perceived all the events in my life.

Reiki is also a great detoxifier and a tool to help overcome traumas and illness, such as the loss of a limb or a stroke, or whether you are confined to a wheelchair or suffer from AIDS, MS and ME.

In other words, if you cannot change your life, reiki will help you change the way you look at it.

An example close to home involved my great niece Rihanna who has autism, a condition that brings on high levels of anxiety, which can be disabling. When she was eleven she was chosen to play the part of Badger in the school play. As the date of the performance loomed I worried that anxiety might get the better of her, so I began sending her weekly reiki. On the night of the play I asked the reiki to start flowing, not just for Rihanna but for the whole cast, that is, for the greatest good of all. The play was a great success. After the performance she walked slowly towards me and I congratulated her on doing a great job.

She looked at me in a somewhat confused state, and said, 'Uncle Brian, I don't know how I did that!'

I just smiled at her, and said, 'Reiki energy is reiki magic.'

She laughed.

Another example of reiki reducing anxiety involved a friend's daughter who always got worked up about flying. Some time before her next flight I sent her a reiki. On their return my friend called and said her daughter had been absolutely amazing on the flight and had no problem, as if she was a different girl.

To sum up, reiki is the greatest friend you can find. It is always there, never lets you down and never leaves you. It is the greatest tool you can have for helping others—including animals. My cat Titch used to seek me out at 8.30 p.m. each evening for a ten-minute reiki, purring away throughout the session. I would use it on her before visiting the vet, a traumatic experience at the best of times. After the reiki she would be calm and Eileen could take her without any distress.

Another significant reiki incident happened on 25 August 2008. It had been a rough night for me —it was too humid and I had not had enough sleep. Feeling drained, after breakfast I sat in the lounge, my back against the front window trying to cool down. As I was nodding off, I heard a loud thud against the window, which woke me with a jolt. I turned around to see a blackbird on the windowsill, seemingly on its last legs. He had obviously flown into the window. Its eyes were closed and it was shaking and swaying, with excretions coming from every orifice. I stood up to face it through the window and began to send it reiki, my arms outstretched, my palms against the window pane, asking for his greatest good at this time with this healing energy. Of course, there are no guarantees of a miracle cure with reiki but it can seemingly happen. Also, if it was the blackbird's time to pass, reiki would ensure a smooth, peaceful transition.

However, after five minutes it suddenly opened its eyes, the excretions stopped and for the next few minutes we stared at each other intently. Then he turned around and flew into the tree in the garden, where he perched on a branch. I continued the reiki, asking for his greatest good and giving thanks to reiki and all who may be helping.

A few minutes later he flew off and I wished him well. I began to wonder whether he would have survived without the healing power of reiki. Who knows?

By this time I had been a reiki master for twelve months. I look back now and realise that it was probably meant to happen, a part of my learning, if you like. The shift in energy vibration from level two to masters level is massive. The incident with the blackbird showed me just how powerful it could be.

But this is not the end of the story. The following August I was getting a little exercise in my garden by pruning a few shrubs, when out of nowhere a blackbird appeared on the fence, not two feet away. He was staring intently at me, so I said, 'Hello,' (as you do!), expecting him to fly off in fright. He didn't budge. I carried on pruning and thinking, how strange. When I moved to put my tools away in the shed he flew off.

That evening I was making an entry in my diary when I noticed the date: 25 August. All the following day, the date kept bugging me. But why? I pulled out the previous year's diary and turned to 25 August. It was the day I had helped the blackbird that crashed into my window.

Coincidence? I think not.

Was it the same blackbird returning to say 'Thank you'? I think so.

If I was offered all the money in the world in exchange for my reiki abilities, I would answer a firm, 'You must be joking.' But if I had been offered the money in 2001 when I became seriously unwell and knew nothing of reiki, I would have taken it, hoping to find answers with it. I now realise that I had to go through the suffering of the last twenty years to learn the true value of reiki healing, and how I needed to lose a lot of wrong thinking in my life.

After six months of reiki healing with Barbara I felt well enough to consider matters other than my own small sphere of illness. I realised that I could make a claim to the Department of Work and Pensions for industrial disease from the chemicals I had ingested. The option that interested me— known as DWP C3—allowed people to claim for injuries incurred while dealing with organophosphorus chemicals. I collated the paperwork to present my case, which included doctors' notes, my own personal notes and cuttings, including an important *Observer* article with the headline "Pollutants Cause Huge Rise in Brain Diseases". The article highlighted the alarming rise in brain diseases, and reproduced statistics showing how rates of dementia had trebled in men, which had been linked to rises in levels of pesticides, industrial effluent, domestic waste, car exhausts and other pollutants. It said that in the late 1970s there were around 3,000 deaths a year from these conditions in England and Wales. By the late 1990s, there were 10,000. The UN estimates that 200,000 people a year die from pesticide exposure. Meanwhile the WHO says one million a year suffer from it.

The causes, the *Observer* article claimed, were commonplace items used in almost every aspect of modern life, from processed food to packaging, from electrical goods to sofa covers, and excessive spraying of food.

In November 2004 my case came up before the tribunal. The rules stated that the claimant had to be told who would be present at the hearing. I was heartened to see that one of the medics would be an allergist, but a week before the due date, they sent a letter saying the allergist had been replaced by a generalist. I thought, this is fishy. The one person who might have understood my condition had been taken off the case. Anyway, I went along and presented my case in front of a judge with a medic sitting either side of him. Then I left the room while they made their judgment.

On returning to the room, the judge said, 'Your claim has to prove that you experience 14% disability before we can make a payment. We've decided to make the award at 20%.'

I thought, that's not brilliant but it proves my point, which is all I wanted.

'However,' he quickly added, 'we're going to take away 15% of the claim for previous and ongoing exposures to chemicals.'

My heart sank.

'Having said that,' he continued, 'I would advise you to continue your claim, not for industrial disease but for industrial injury, that is, an accident at work.'

I went home and considered all that the judge had said. On one hand it was disappointing that my claim had been passed over for not reaching the 14% threshold for industrial disease, but on the other I was pleased that he had confirmed that I was subject to further ongoing environmental exposure, which was central to my case. I may have been disappointed on the day but I knew his comments could be helpful further down the line.

I saw little point in trying to claim for an industrial injury, but I did claim for Disability

Living Allowance for my general disabilities. I won the lower level of mobility assessment and middle rate for the psychological effects and fatigue. To this day I am regularly assessed to ensure I meet the criteria. In 2019 that criteria was tightened, so much so that thousands of people had their benefits taken away, which in some cases led to suicides. I was lucky, the medical assessor could see I was still disabled, and allowed the support to continue. There is always a danger that when a specialist condition such as mine is assessed by nurses with no background or knowledge of OP poisoning, they may not be aware of the crippling symptoms, many of which are not immediately apparent. Consequently I make sure I am genned up on the subject before they come to see me.

But of course these assessments are extremely stressful situations in themselves requiring lots of physical, mental and emotional energy, which always takes its toll on my health, and invariably leads to a relapse.

Victims of ME–CFS will tell you we cannot tolerate even small amounts of stress, due, I believe, to the lack of stress hormones we have or are capable of producing. Remember the build-up of acetylcholine due to organophosphorus poisoning. Acetylcholine is a major on switch. We cannot relax; we get irritable, anxious, sleepless, severely fatigued and depressed—all symptoms of OP poisoning and ME–CFS.

CHAPTER 6

Forget injuries, never forget kindness – Confucius

On a post-Christmas shopping trip in January 2010 I slipped on the tiled floor of the Millgate shopping centre in Bury and broke my right hip. My first thought was that if this is an open fracture I am in serious trouble because of my aversion to anaesthetics and all the drugs that go with an operation. In my situation most people would be desperate to get to hospital (that is, somewhere where they will get some help) but I was praying that I wouldn't be taken because of all the chemicals, and where I could be made to feel worse (at best). Such is the predicament of someone with hypersensitivity to chemicals. I couldn't get off the floor, so I had no choice but to be taken to hospital and, of course, the doctors wanted to operate under general anaesthetic. I explained that I could not allow that because I knew the anaesthetic may finish me off. I showed them my medic alert bracelet, which explained my condition with a number to ring.

I spent twelve days in hospital while they decided what to do with me. One day as I lay on the bed in an atmosphere permeated by pharmaceuticals and medications, my hypersensitivity could pick up the effects of the anaesthetic emanating from the patient in the next bed who had just returned from surgery—so much so that it put me out for four hours.

I remember a male paramedic questioning the wisdom of my refusal to have the operation. His sympathies lay with Eileen.

He asked, 'How is your wife going to look after you if you return home with a broken hip?'

I took his question with a pinch of salt and suggested politely that he read up on OP poisoning and its effects on susceptible people. I told him to buy the book *Stop the 21st Century Killing You* by Dr Baillie-Hamilton.

I also recall one evening in hospital the drugs nurse wheeling her trolley around the ward. When she got to my bed she picked up my chart and had an unbelievable look of puzzlement on her face.

She said, 'Where's your drug chart?'

'I am drug intolerant,' I replied. 'I cannot go near them.'

'This cannot be right. No one comes onto a fracture ward and has no pain relief, it's not possible.'

'I'm afraid it is,' I said.

I then told her about reiki and offered to send her an absent distant healing using my symbols. She agreed to accept it and I sent it that night timed for when her head hit the pillow.

The following day, she said, 'Thank you. I haven't slept like that for twenty years.'

'Do yourself a favour,' I said, 'and buy yourself a book on reiki!'

My consultant offered to send me home with a hospital bed to undergo a period of traction in an effort to heal the hip. I was happy about that but the ward sister was sure that the bed would not fit into my bungalow. What was my prognosis? They said the hip would eventually heal but that it was likely one leg would be shorter than the other. They were right: my right leg healed 3–4 centimetres shorter than my left.

As I left hospital a medic asked me, 'What are you going to do for pain relief?'

I replied, 'Reiki!'

Of course, the medics thought I was barking mad. I arrived home and eased myself into the bed. Forty-eight hours later I was in agony. The pain relief that I had absorbed from the hospital environment must have worked its way out of my system. There was no other plausible explanation. I was now on my own, in excruciating pain, completely immobile, facing the prospect of being bedbound for months and unable even to use the shower. Between January and July Eileen had to do everything for me, including making and bringing me all my meals.

After what seemed like an age I felt stronger and the hospital sent a physiotherapist to my home to help with rehabilitation.

At this time I was also doing four hours of self-reiki healings every day and getting monthly acupuncture sessions. I cannot imagine how I would have coped without the healings, or indeed where I would have ended up without Eileen's help.

CHAPTER 7

That's (my) life

*Kindness is a language that the deaf can hear and
the blind can see* – Mark Twain

I regard myself as the two-hour man because that's my approximate limit of energy at any one time. In between those two hours of 'activity' I rest, but I can't relax like other people might: putting your feet up and watching TV. For me even that can be too taxing. I can't even read, and am in bed by 10 p.m. each evening. I have to retreat into an almost meditative state to regain my sense of well-being. I can sometimes reiki myself to help return to normal life. If I didn't have the reiki I don't believe I would have carried on. In my darkest moments I can't see any way out of my depression. I become bereft of physical, emotional and mental strength. The psychological impact of that is tremendous.

Since Eileen and I parted, I have had to do all my own cleaning, shopping and cooking. I have to be careful where I go whenever I do venture out. I am always on red alert. I never had the confidence to learn to drive so I get a taxi to the shops because I can't take public transport with all the passengers who have chemicals on their clothing. My condition took away all my confidence but reiki is beginning to bring it back. I have learned that everything has an energy, which is as unique as one's fingerprints. With reiki you vibrate at a higher energy and feel more empathetic towards the world.

Having said that I reckon I have about a third of the energy of a normal person, that is, the person I once was. Consequently I have to use it wisely and save it up to do one activity per day. When I have to do housework, shopping and cooking, I have little stamina left for anything else.

All my food has to be organic otherwise the following day I have terrible stomach problems. My diet is necessarily limited because I also have IBS. After I achieved reiki masters level I went off meat, primarily because I didn't like the idea of eating anything that had lived. I kept looking at the neighbourhood cats and thinking, *No*! I believe this change in my values came from reiki's spiritual side that has encouraged me to think about the world in ways I hadn't considered before. Consequently I get all my protein from beans, eggs, some cheese, fruit and vegetables. My staples are organic rice and whole spelt. All my water has to be filtered for both drinking and cooking. If I drink tap water directly I feel terrible. Six weeks after I started using a water filter I noticed an improvement.

Sport and music are my two passions, but if there's a football match on TV I have to prepare myself for the match, so I let something else go on that day to build up my strength just to watch the game. If I'm in a relapse period I can only manage the first half of the game and have to record the rest to watch the following day.

Most people will say that what I'm living is not a life but just an existence. If I did not have the reiki, I would probably agree with them.

Common to people with my condition is the inability to properly regulate my body temperature. People coming to my house may feel it a bit chilly, but no matter what kind of condition I'm in, I can only run the boiler for two hours a day, and permanently set the thermostat at 15 degrees C. During a summer heatwave or a cold snap in winter I have great difficulty adjusting my temperature. If I am bedbound all I require is a jacket around me, just enough to get what I call 'naturally warm'. Even then I am still using the ceiling fan to keep a draught of air in the room. I experience these swings of heat and cold because my hypothalamus (the region of the brain that controls the sensory nerves) is damaged. Consequently I keep waking up during the night because I'm either too hot or too cold. I cannot sleep *in* a bed because I get too hot. I have to sleep *on top of* the bedding with a jacket over me. Yet if I put on an extra jacket I boil up. The hot/cold predicament seems to me to be the distinction between people with depression (who have my utmost sympathy) and people with ME. ME sufferers all have body temperature irregularities, which became a major feature of my illness after the collapse of the court case in 2001: four days and nights without sleep or food and swinging between red hot and freezing cold, and shivering violently as if I was having a fit. The tail end of that horror show continued for weeks. The situation got me down and I began to wonder would I have to live like this for the rest of my life?

The only thing that could reach me at this time was reiki. As I have said, exercising reiki on myself helps, but the effects are far greater if I get another reiki master to send me the healing. That takes the edge off. If I'm in a good phase and receive a healing I get a real lift. It's been my saviour. It doesn't only heal *my* pain, lifts my spirits and aids sleep, but I've also used it on my sister and her children and I can see how they have subsequently taken great strides forward in their lives.

Lately I have found that suitable music, played at the right time of day and according to my mood and health, is a great comfort. I was a child of the sixties—the Beatles, Fleetwood Mac, Bob Dylan, the Rolling Stones and all that hippy music was the soundtrack to my youth. Dylan and Lennon were great favourites of mine who were not only singing pop ditties, but also wrote great songs with deeper messages. Nowadays when I have my bad times on the bed I put on Classic FM to relax.

One year, to celebrate ME Day (yes, there is such a thing—12 May), a musical trio from the BBC Philharmonic came round to the house. Later they sent a journalist who asked me what my favourite piece of music was. It didn't take me long to pick "The Lark Ascending" by Ralph Vaughan Williams, which really hits the spot. In recent years I have discovered the Royal Marine Band's version of the emotive "The Ashokan Farewell". While restful music can help me relax, if I rest too long I go down and down and have to tune in to livelier radio stations to bring me back up.

Any change to my environment can have devastating effects on me. In June 2005 I got very ill as a direct consequence of a neighbour building a house extension. The chemicals he was using (probably formaldehyde, amongst others) affected me so badly that my body temperature regulator went haywire and I spent three weeks in a terrible state; I could only wear a pair of tracksuit bottoms and nothing else. The ceiling fan was never off, and I only slept about three hours each night. My respiration was severely affected to the extent that I didn't know where I was. I was also unable to shower during this three-week period, and lost a stone in weight.

Around this time I was due to be reassessed for Incapacity Benefit. The official claim had to be completed by my GP, on which he wrote, "Principle effects are multiple environmental sensitivities [which] result in symptoms equivalent to severe chronic fatigue syndrome—chronic anxiety—lowered mood from pesticide toxicity at work."

Well, he was right about the 'environmental sensitivities'!

I was constantly scouring the newspapers for stories about people who had similar experiences. In 1998 a former draughtsman who worked for the Duke of Northumberland in the print room at Alnwick Castle was awarded £100,000 compensation after being exposed to excessive quantities of ammonia. The defendants (the trustees of the ninth duke) claimed his illness, which initially showed itself in flu-like symptoms, was psychological. He became so sensitive to chemicals that even the smell of a woman's perfume made him ill. His condition worsened to such an extent that exposure to paint, creosote, crop spray, household polishes and sheep dip left him housebound. Clearly he discovered what I had already deduced: dioxins found in everyday objects can be deleterious to one's health.

I felt so strongly about the subject that in June 2008 I wrote a letter to the *Manchester Evening News*, which was reprinted under the headline "Hidden Danger", reproduced below.

"With regard to the story of people being burned with fungicides used as anti-mould agents in sofas. I believe it is only the tip of the iceberg with regard to chemical exposures and chronic ill health.

In 2004 I was diagnosed with brain function impairment (commonly termed ME) and received a disability pension for it. I was told my disability was caused by chemical exposure at work and also from a neighbouring farm.

In 1988 the government passed a law making it compulsory to treat soft furnishings, including bedding and mattresses, with powerful chemicals as fire retardants. Research done at Manchester University has shown that certain genetic types are very vulnerable to these chemicals, they lack an enzyme called paraoxonase, which is the body's first line of defence. Many scientific reports have linked pesticides and ill health, including ME, Parkinson's disease, cancers, IBS and others, plus they have also been linked with depression/anxiety and suicides.

This damage to the nervous system can take years and is long-term and incurable. My local council tell me they spray the borough with weed-killer but you are breathing it and taking it home on your clothing if you are out and about at the time of spraying.

Talk of green issues is futile while we are being exposed to damaging chemicals."

I referred to certain genetic types being more vulnerable to chemicals, by which I meant that I must have been susceptible from childhood. Living close to the paper mill certainly didn't help.

In her book *It's Mitochondria, Not Hypochondria* Dr Sarah Myhill lays out the case for identifying underlying causes of health problems, especially the 'diseases of civilisation' with which we are beset in the West. Essentially her contention is that there is a genetic link that makes certain people susceptible. We get all our mitochondria from the mother not the father. Curiously my sister's daughter Phillipa has been diagnosed with the same condition as me. My nephew Brandon has been diagnosed with ADHD and my other niece Rihanna has been diagnosed with autism. This convinces me that there is a genetic link. Once the damage has been done to the gene it will be passed down the female line and can emerge in a variety of conditions.

In 2014 I requested genotyping for a paraoxonase in site 55 and 192, the damaged genes which I believed made me more susceptible to OP poisoning. My objective was to identify a physical link between my genes and my susceptibilities. The hospital's response was to dismiss my enquiry, having regarded the possibility of a link with my condition as "a very thin association". Instead they referred me to the department of occupational health. And yes, you've guessed it. They also refused to see me.

A research document called The Scope Project, produced by The Centre for Occupational and Environmental Health at Manchester University examined whether certain people were more susceptible to developing ill health following exposure to organophosphates. The project showed an inability to detoxify quickly enough. The full report appeared in *The Lancet* and supported the idea that some people may be at particular risk from working with OPs. Some of the people who took part in the study were able to access the C3 industrial disease pension—the one I was denied. Not such a thin association after all.

CHAPTER 8

The world is changed by your example, not by your opinion – Paulo Coelho

I have always had a passion for helping people or animals. When I reached reiki masters level I was told I could send my healing anywhere in the world. I was sceptical, to say the least. The practitioner, Karen Barlow, said, 'Try it and see.'

I started with the family.

On one occasion my first niece, Melanie, had a bad dose of flu so I said I would send her the healing. The next day I called her and told her to lie down and get comfortable. I did my signs (now I don't need to do the signs, I just *think* the healing and it goes). Before I put the phone down at 1.30 p.m. I asked her to ring me once she had had a five-minute rest. By 2.15 p.m. she hadn't rung back. As it was my first remote reiki healing, I hoped she was okay and was mildly worried what might have happened to her. At 3 p.m. the phone rang; it was Melanie.

I said, 'Are you okay?'

Rather blearily, she said, 'I've just woken up.'

'Well that's amazing. It really does travel! Call me in half an hour when you've come round.'

She did and said she felt fine, but I was knocked out at the power I had transmitted.

On another occasion (this time when I was at the house) Melanie's young son Ben was having a bit of a strop. He lay up against his mother on the couch. I did my healing and before I knew it they had both fallen asleep.

I went back a week later.

Ryan, the older son, opened the door and, with a chuckle, said, 'Hello, Uncle Brian, have you come to put Ben to sleep?'

I said, 'Ryan, I'm not a vet!'

I realised then that this reiki was something else. I know most people will say the so-called power is all in the mind, but I don't care because I know it works. And so does everyone who has benefitted from this unique energy healing.

By 2005 I had become overweight, reaching sixteen stone at my heaviest. Over the next two years I lost three stone, which I put down to the reiki clearing out toxins and other distractions from my life that were doing me harm.

I also added another unconventional therapy to my treatment plan.

In 2006 I was flicking through the Yellow Pages (remember that?) looking for complementary treatments for allergies when I discovered another holistic treatment that claimed to help people relax and make them more able to face the world: mora therapy. Karen Barlow explained what was involved: no more than sitting in a comfy chair opposite a computer screen and holding onto two brass handles while placing my bare feet on a brass plate. She said the machine would read every organ in the body, right down to the cells and nervous system.

The mora ethos states that we have to be in balance to be well; the machine tells Karen what's out of balance. Everyone has their own oscillation spectrum, so the therapy uses endogenic oscillations that correspond to one's physiological condition. Once this information is electronically processed and fed back, it is possible to change the physical and physiological conditions in the body and to initiate the healing processes. The mora machine also shows if your chemical allergies are increasing due to ongoing exposures. In fact the sensitivities are always heavily increased in spring and autumn when crop spraying is widely undertaken.

On my first visit Karen said she would test for sensitivity to chemicals. My readings for formaldehyde and a certain pesticide was 90+% sensitivity (less than 5% is reasonable).

She looked at the readings and said, 'No wonder you're not well!'

Now, back to reiki... I had been attuned to level 1 in 2003 and Barbara said that I will know when the time was right to progress to level 2 and later become a reiki master practitioner. That time was upon me. In 2007 I woke up one morning and it immediately dawned on me that I wanted to reach the next level.

That's when all the weird stuff started happening.

Apart from football, rugby and cricket, I've always loved horse racing, both for the sporting aspect and also because I like a flutter at the weekend on the big races. Both my grandfathers were not averse to putting a few hard-earned shillings on the horses.

A month after I achieved masters level in reiki I woke up with a song from the sixties buzzing in my head. The same thing happened the following morning. And again on the third day. I was looking at the Friday evening paper to check the horses racing in the weekend's race meetings when I came across a horse whose name linked to the song that had been buzzing in my head. I thought, amused at the very idea, maybe a higher power is trying to tell me something and I should listen to it by placing a bet. Surely not. I didn't. The horse won at 10–1.

A fortnight later I got another song in my head called "Streetlife". I looked at the weekend's races in the paper. As if I'd planted it, there was a horse running with the same name. I put a fiver on. It won at 4–1.

Once was surely a coincidence; twice was spooky. I wondered if it might have been one of my grandads sending me messages. I called the reiki practitioner and she laughed and said she had heard of this kind of thing happening before.

'Now that you've reached masters level the vibrations are far stronger, which can put you in contact with all sorts of things. If I were you I would accept it as a gift for all the reiki you have done for other people without charging a penny.'

Before the July York races I got another tune in my head and spotted a horse in the field that directly correlated to the song. I couldn't keep it to myself and had to tell Eileen what was going on. She thought I was loopy. I went to the bookies: £10 each way at 11–1.

I came home and watched the race with a very sceptical Eileen. My horse led the race from start to finish.

Where were these messages coming from? Was someone building me up for a massive fall by tempting me to place a large bet and then lose?

One day I walked to my sister's place, a ten-minute walk away. Halfway there I came across some kids playing football in the street.

A little boy came up to me, and said, 'Mister, do you want to buy a leaflet?'

'What's it about?'

From behind his back he pulled an advertising flyer for a local taxi firm. He had obviously picked it up from the gutter.

I played along with the cheeky fellow and asked, 'How much?'

'Ten pence.'

'How much for two?'

'Twenty pence.'

I said, 'Go on then.'

I returned home with a flyer in my pocket.

Eileen said, 'Something strange happened while you were gone. A taxi drove into the close, parked up, and sat there for ten minutes before driving off without picking up a passenger. Fifteen minutes later he did the same. And then again a third time.

I agreed that was very strange. Somewhat excited, I told Eileen about the cheeky little boy and the taxi leaflet.

She said, 'Now you think this is a message about another horse, don't you?'

(Even though Eileen was by now a level 2 reiki healer, she was still sceptical.)

I said, 'Well, let's find out, shall we?'

I got the *Manchester Evening News* and noticed a horse called "Tony the Taxi" that was running in a minor meeting. The form suggested it had absolutely no chance. It came nowhere. I didn't place a bet, I just looked at it as another form of communication or psychic growth.

They say some people develop psychic ability because of the higher vibrations to which their brain is attuned. I link this to the doctor who said that OP damage is an increased form of sensitivity. It's there for everyone but you have to reach a certain level of vibration to be able to pick it up. I liken it to the improvements in radio technology over the years: we went from AM to shortwave then FM to digital. If you are not attuned to the frequencies, you cannot pick up the signal.

By now I had accepted that messages were being left for me everyday, it was just a question of finding them. By this time I could not believe there was such a thing as coincidence, it was a matter of interpreting messages left for me. Each time I put on the TV or radio, I would notice a recurring word, name or phrase and a theme would emerge.

One day I was listening to the sports news on BBC Radio 5 during which a reporter was interviewing a golfer. It seemed innocuous enough but after a couple of days I felt that somebody was trying to tell me something. Then TV showed a programme about golf. Soon after I took the bus to go to the organic food shop, and when I had reached Radcliffe library I looked up and saw a guy getting on the bus with a set of golf clubs slung over his shoulder. That in itself would have been remarkable, but after the earlier signs I knew something was brewing. I had also been receiving the number 17 in various ways but I couldn't yet see the connection. A couple of days before a big race my sister was looking through the paper for the runners and riders. She saw a horse called "Just A Par", even though she didn't recognise the significance of the name, I noticed the direct connection to golf. So where did the number 17 come into it? The horse was not number 17 so I dropped the idea and decided I was creating something out of nothing.

Saturday came and I put the TV on around 2 p.m. when the sports coverage was building up to the big 3.30 p.m. race. The reporter was interviewing the winner of the previous race.

'Gee, Sean,' he said, 'that was a hell of a ride for a seventeen-year-old.'

I went cold. I looked at my watch which showed the big race at Sandown was due to start in an hour. Surely Sean Bowen wasn't riding Just a Par. I grabbed the paper and looked at the race. I was stunned. Yes, it was amazing. For ten minutes I ummed and ahhed. *Do it*, I thought. I ran down to the bookies and bet £10 each way on Just a Par at 16–1. From the bookies I went directly to my sister's place and explained the connection between golf and the number 17 and told everyone about the cryptic messages that a certain horse was going to win a big race. Verna and her whole family got excited, everyone was now gathered around the TV.

They set off. Just a Par was stuck at the back for most of the race. With three fences to go, we heard the excited commentator say, 'Making rapid headway from the back is Just a Par.'

The horse approached the last fence in third place but seemed to fly over the jump and ran away from the field. Everyone in the house was left staring at the TV, mouths wide open.

I won £230. I felt a strange kind of power, but not the power to win at whim. Knowing that I had the ability to interpret these signs was a greater gift to me than the money, and I always share my good fortune.

Of course, the horse bets didn't always win, but usually came in second or third, so I didn't lose on my each-way bets.

I'm more used to making law-of-averages bets, which involved studying the form of horses and football teams before laying a sensible each-way bet. For instance, I would monitor how long it had been since Manchester United had a 1–0 home win. The law of averages told me that they were probably due that score if they hadn't won 1–0 at Old Trafford for eight or nine games, in which case it was probably worth a bet.

In 2015 Man United were playing an evening match away against Newcastle, and the game was due to be broadcast live on TV. They had not had an away 0–1 win in fourteen games. Before the match, MUTV interviewed Ashley Young and the reporter mentioned that it was well over twelve months since he had scored. I considered the law of averages once again. It would have been a hell of a win to bet on Young to score in a 0–1 away win, so I lay two bets: £25 on United winning 0–1 (at 5–1), and £5 on Ashley Young to be the first scorer (at 75–1).

The bookie looked at me askance, and must have thought, *Easy money.*

After ninety minutes there was no score. In extra time Wayne Rooney made a last ditch attack that was fumbled away by the defender. The ball skewed away from him and across an empty penalty area. The first player to the ball? Ashley Young, who side-footed it into the net. There was still another minute of extra time, which I watched, hardly believing what had happened. United won 0–1. I won £520.

In the run-up to another Man Utd game, this time against Leeds, I had been getting messages about the blind. I was washing-up one day when a delivery driver tried to deliver a parcel to a neighbour, who was out. I took in the parcel and noticed the label was from Guide Dogs for the Blind. At this time Eileen was working at Remploy, the disabled employment placement service, and she had befriended a thalidomide girl who was married to a blind man. Then it dawned on me that one of the Man U substitutes was Kieran Richardson—the thalidomide girl's surname was Richardson. The problem was that Richardson did not start too many games, so the likelihood of him scoring was slim.

I went to the bookies on the Saturday and asked for the odds on the game. Despite the long odds I put the bet on for Richardson to score the first goal. I watched the build-up to the match and as the teams were lined up in the tunnel waiting to come onto the pitch, the commentator announced that there had been a late change. Giggs was injured and Richardson was taking his place. During the match a midfielder got the ball to Rooney who tried to go around the keeper, but the ball flew into no-man's land and Richardson slotted the ball home. The game ended 1–1 but I was still convinced the link had been made—and it made me some money.

My explanation for all these messages is that reiki is all about balance, so even though I had plenty of successful days, my good fortune needed to be balanced. Nevertheless I look at these sporting situations as my apprenticeship towards receiving messages on a more profound level.

One of these messages I received for a lady called Louise who worked in the Village Greens organic shop. She was hobbling around due to a problem with the ligaments in her leg. She said that the NHS just couldn't seem to heal it.

'I'm on permanent painkillers, which is far from ideal,' she said.

I offered to send her some reiki healing. 'You've got nothing to lose,' I said.

She agreed.

That night I sent her the healing. A week later I was in the shop and saw Louise on her pushbike. She pointed at me and, evidently pleased at the improvement in her leg, said, 'You are a miracle worker.'

'Please don't call me that,' I said, but secretly I was very pleased for her.

Another time I met a woman called Anabelle who mentioned that she had recently been diagnosed with ME. I told her that, as a fellow sufferer, she had my heartfelt sympathy, and the only treatment I had found to help was reiki. She asked if I would mind helping her. Of course not.

I sent her some healing that night. Next time I saw her she said that she had never slept so soundly. Her mother, who I had never met and whose name I did not know, had recently died. I said that I could ask her mother if she had any messages for Anabelle. She probably thought, *I'll just humour him.*

I came home and sent the healing. Next morning there was a voice in my head that uttered the name 'Val'.

The name meant nothing to me and I had no reason to connect the message with Anabelle. The next time I went to the shop, she mentioned that she felt so much better.

Tentatively she asked, 'What did you learn about my mother?'

I said that I was unsure; however, I was made aware of a name: Val.

She exclaimed, 'That was my mum's name.'

Afterwards I was asked to connect with her brother. The following morning another random name came to me: Mathew, her brother's name.

I had by now accepted that the reiki energy had been integrated into me. I believed that my life was preordained because before I became ill I was an everyday guy, never thinking there could be anything beyond my life. If I had never suffered the way I did I would never have been aware of this other power. I do believe that true learning about reiki healing has to come from the heart and from real suffering otherwise the practitioner would remain consumed by the material world.

I told Anabelle about mora therapy, which piqued her interest. She wanted to try it so she picked me up one day and we drove to the treatment centre in Todmorden together. As soon as I got into the car I picked up on her energy. In fact, I think we picked up on each other's energy because we never stopped talking the whole time, there and back; it was like electricity.

In my thirties, before I met Eileen, I used to know a woman called Sandra, who subsequently died of non-Hodgkin's lymphoma. Nothing took off between her and I but I was left with the feeling that I was meant to help her in some way. This was before I got involved in reiki.

Now we scroll ahead to Christmas morning, 1999. At that time we still had one of the old, heavy televisions that had a lip around the screen. That morning I noticed a card pushed into the bottom of the screen. Eileen swore that she hadn't placed it there. Maybe it had fallen somehow, she suggested. But that was not possible. Was that Sandra...?

In 2007, for three mornings in a row, I woke up very emotional with thoughts of Sandra. It was strange because I hadn't seen her in years. I then bumped into a mutual friend who I asked if she had seen Sandra lately. No. Two weeks later, after a spell being bedbound, I took a stroll to the barber's and, walking back along a quiet road, I saw a lady walking towards me. From fifty metres away she looked like Sandra, or at least like her as an older woman. I planned to say hello when our paths crossed but she did not acknowledge me and kept looking straight ahead. She looked unwell and I figured that, if it was her, she hadn't recognised me. After thirty metres I looked back and saw the woman had also stopped and was looking back at me.

Still uncertain about the identity of the woman, I made enquiries to see if Sandra lived locally. No.

Some time later I bumped into the mutual friend again, who said, 'I'm glad I've seen you because I remember you asked me about Sandra.'

Before she went any further, I said, 'I think I saw her.'

'No,' she said, 'You couldn't have, she passed in 1997.'

I was shocked but put the similarity of the woman on the street down to a lookalike.

I was telling Karen at the mora centre about the incident who suggested I call Mr Mack, a dowser in Brighton, who might be able to shed some light on the episode. He said that often if people who were highly drugged pass, they can become a confused earthbound spirit, i.e., not fully passed over. But because of the reiki they would notice you with some kind of ring of light around your head emanating from the higher vibrations.

'Is there anything you can do?' I asked.

He said that he would work on it that evening and suggested I call back on Saturday morning. He wasn't trying to swindle me because he charged nothing for his rather unique services. He suggested a charity to which I could make a donation if I wished. After the substantial winnings on the sports bets I had already set up two direct debits: one to Guide Dogs for the Blind, and one for Save the Children.

Thursday night as I went to bed I sent Sandra a reiki with Mr Mack's help. *If you get this let me know*. At 1 a.m. I woke up and involuntarily let out a terrible scream. As I calmed down I felt someone lightly hug me around the waist, and then they were gone. I told her that I was pleased the energy worked and to send me three signals to verify the contact.

The following morning as I was having breakfast I decided to put on the TV. I usually watched a news update but that morning the TV was tuned to a radio station. As I turned up the sound, a song called "I'll Carry You Home" was playing. The words kept resonating in my brain. Wasn't that what I had just helped Sandra to do? I set off to pick up some shopping, thinking, *Is this the first signal*? When I reached the shopping mall I went into a CD shop and asked them who sang "I'll Carry You Home". They said it was by James Blunt from his new album called "All the Lost Souls". I couldn't speak. A lost soul being carried home. I couldn't have made it up.

However, I knew from past experience there was usually one word that signals a communication verification and as yet that hadn't happened. I didn't have to wait long.

I needed to go into WH Smith for some stationery. It was a Saturday so the place was packed. As I entered, a young boy's voice boomed out above the din, 'No, Mum, I want to go to John Thompson's.' I thought, OMG, Sandra's surname was Thompson. Was Sandra going to use her surname as the signal? I would soon get my answer. On arriving home I made a hot drink and switched on the kitchen radio. A song was playing called "Love on your Side". I hadn't a clue about the name of the band. At the end of the song the DJ said, 'That was "Love on your Side" by The Thompson Twins.'

My immediate thoughts were, *that's two Thompsons in no time at all.* I began to wonder how she would send the third signal. Within twenty minutes I had my answer. I was chopping some vegetables when I heard the letterbox ping. The mail was not usually delivered at that time of the afternoon so I went to see what had been delivered. What was on the porch floor? *Thompson's Local Directory.*

I rang Mack and he chuckled. 'I've heard of this kind of thing before,' he said, 'that was her saying thank you before leaving.'

In 2012 I was put in touch with a woman called Ruby, a nurse and fellow ME victim. One day I offered to send her a reiki. She had never heard of such a thing but she agreed to accept it. Next day we spoke again and she said she had slept really well the previous night. I sent reiki healing to her a couple more times as she was clearly receptive to it. In passing, Ruby mentioned that she had been very close to her grandmother who had passed two years previously, and had recently been getting upset about it. I told her that the next time I send her a reiki I will ask if her grandmother was there and if she had any messages for her. I expect she thought, *Sure you will!* What came through over the next few weeks amazed even me.

When I receive clairaudient messages (hearing what others cannot hear) they tend to arrive as I'm waking up in the morning when I am at my most relaxed and receptive. On this particular morning I got a vision of a hammer with the specific date 21 May. Even though the message meant nothing to me, I called Ruby and mentioned it to her.

She let out a startled cry, and said, 'It feels like you're stalking me, you can't possibly know this.'

'What is it?'

She said she had gone to court six months before with a woman friend whose husband had been abusing her. She remembered the case occurred in late spring. She opened her diary and confirmed the court date was 21 May when the husband was accused of attacking her friend with a hammer.

'How did you know that?' she asked.

I said, 'I know I can't know this, but I do and have to pass it on to you.'

Time went on and I sent another reiki.

She called and asked, 'Has anything come through?'

I said, 'It's not like using a telephone, I can't ask for a message. I just have to wait for it to come to me.'

One morning I woke late at 10.30 a.m. In a soft tone I heard a voice say, 'Frank Wilson.'

The name meant nothing to me and I wondered once more if it had something to do with Ruby.

I rang her and she screamed down the phone, 'No, no, I don't believe it! Yesterday I got a phone call from my brother who is into Northern Soul music. He wanted to buy a rare limited edition release, which meant going into Nottingham to buy a copy. He didn't have a car so he asked if I would take him. Anyway, I picked him up at 10.30 a.m. and we went to the shop. What struck me as I entered was that on one wall was a full-size picture of a soul singer called Frank Wilson, who had released the record my brother wanted to buy.'

I was astonished at the accuracy of the message, and said, 'I believe your grandmother was probably in the car with you because that's the precise time when I got the message.'

That was enough to send shivers down both our spines, but there would be a final message that flabbergasted us both.

Some time later I was talking to Ruby, and she asked, 'Any more messages?'

'Funny you should say that. I did get a message from a voice saying, "Sunderland and money". Does that mean anything to you?'

With astonishment in her voice, she said, 'I am right now sitting at my kitchen table and have just received a cheque from my ex-husband who lives in Sunderland.'

Later, another name came to me after I had sent a distant healing to Sophia Mirza, a woman I had never met but whose demise was the first official death from ME–chronic fatigue syndrome. It may seem an unusual thing to do to send reiki to someone who had been deceased for some time, but I had been reading a lot about this brave soldier and thought it would do no harm to express my solidarity with her.

A few days later, as I was waking up one morning, a quiet voice said to me, 'Dr David Hanson.' My sister Googled his name and it turned out that he was a roboticist in Japan who had made a 'female' robot. But where was the link to Sophia? The name of the robot: Sophia.

I asked the deceased Sophia if there was a way she could message me three times to confirm she had received my reiki. I put the TV on channel 3 that happened to be showing *This Morning* where the presenters were talking to a man with a lady sat next to him. The man was Dr David Hansen who was sitting next to Sophia the robot. This was the signal I had been hoping for.

I realise that if I started talking like this to my GP he would probably send me for psychiatric evaluation. But I choose to believe the evidence before me.

I also wondered why paranormal events, clairvoyance and telepathy, for example, were kept out of the public eye, in much the same way that chemical victims were.

A good example of this occurred one day, around fifteen years ago, when I was listening to a national radio station which aired a phone-in programme on people's personal experiences of unexplained events. I was a regular listener to the two-hour programme which was a huge success and always inundated with calls, but it only lasted for a few months and disappeared overnight without warning. I wondered why would they take the show off the air. It felt to me that the powers that be didn't want people being educated about what was out there. If you look, maybe the establishment don't want the materialistic gravy train being derailed by a more spiritual way of thinking, and more importantly, acting. Food for thought.

At first I thought I must be going crazy. We're all brought up to believe clairvoyance and any kind of extrasensory perception is the devil's work. When it first starting happening to me it freaked me out and made me extremely uneasy. But the more I read about reiki the more I learned that clairvoyance can come to certain healers. For some reason it came to me. Now I accept I'm not going mad and that reiki, with all its wondrous powers, is a higher form of energy.

CHAPTER 9

If you want to be a rebel, be kind

For most of my life I would never have dreamed of tackling the seemingly huge task of writing a book. But now that it's done I must say that it has helped imbue me with the confidence that has been missing in my life for so long. When I look around at fellow ME–CFS sufferers I realise how they have been robbed of a full life too because of who they were born to or the neighbourhoods in which they were born and lived.

ME damages the stress response. My hypersensitivity does not mean that I am merely sensitised to a certain chemical or situation—no, I am sensitised to *all* chemicals because my sensory nerves are damaged. If I am subjected to certain chemicals during the day I am only good for laying on the bed. My breathing goes shallow and I have to force myself to almost mechanically inhale and exhale until I get over the trauma.

Some sufferers have great sensitivity to light, which means curtains remain closed during the day. It makes you aware of having to control systems in the body that it should be regulating naturally, and which most people take for granted. To illustrate these symptoms I will highlight two—admittedly serious—high profile ME–CFS cases to underline the debilitating effects of the disease and the medical profession's far from ideal response.

British woman Sophia Mirza—the same Sophia to whom I later sent reiki—died aged thirty-two in 2006. Her last years were truly horrific, during which time her five senses became hypersensitive. Her room had to be completely blacked-out and she wore eye pads as any form of light burned into her. Noise too was unbearable, even the sound of a voice. She could not bear to be touched for the same reason, even though she craved the comfort of human touch. She was unable to have either a bath or a hair wash as water magnified her symptoms. She lay permanently on her right side in an attempt to minimise the pain. She had, for most of this time, been unable to speak, unable to read or write, listen to the radio or have any electrical gadgets in her room, and no visitors, for fear of exacerbating her condition. Sophia refused drugs and on one occasion both the social services and the police took it into their heads to kick the door down and drag her off to a psychiatric hospital, 'for her own good' no doubt. With the help of a solicitor her mother managed to get her released after two weeks. The stress of that experience set her back terribly. She died a cruel death with doctors unable or unwilling to care for and treat this misunderstood illness.

Hers was the first official death from ME–chronic fatigue syndrome, which was a major breakthrough for those of us who know it to be a physical condition. The neuropathologist who gave evidence at her inquest said that Sophia's spinal cord showed inflammation caused by dorsal root ganglionitis, a clear physical manifestation of the disease, and something many medics refuse to accept.

Another patient who suffered tremendously was Lynn Gilderdale from East Sussex. Her symptoms began aged fourteen after she had the BCG vaccine. She became ill and within a couple of weeks her life and health were never to be the same. She struggled on until her death aged thirty-one. Lynn was in so much pain and distress that she begged her mother to help her die. She experienced fits like clockwork at 6 p.m. every evening. To test the legitimacy of her illness, psychiatrists put her in a room with no lights, windows or clocks to see whether she relied on the psychological trigger of seeing a clock reach 6 p.m. before faking her fit. Of course, nothing changed, she still had her fit at the same time. Her mother

Kay also went through hell—watching her daughter suffer and cry out for help is more than any mother can take, so when she found Lynn attempting to kill herself, she helped her daughter take a fatal overdose. Kay Gilderdale, who later wrote an excellent book called *One Last Goodbye*, was later cleared of assisting her daughter to commit suicide.

I view these two young women as spirit warriors for the cause of ME–CFS sufferers everywhere. They did not deserve the disdain and disrespect they got. I believe there is a common link between the two women and most suffers of ME–CFS (including myself) in the effect of the disease on the autonomic nervous system. The first set, called preganglionic neurons, originates in the brainstem or the spinal cord, and the second set, called ganglion cells or postganglionic neurons, lies outside the central nervous system in collections of nerve cells called autonomic ganglia. The HSE MS17 document that identified the dangers of OP pesticides identified these areas as sites of damage in the body caused by direct or indirect exposure to organophosphates. In my case this originated in my ongoing exposure to a neighbouring farm during the period 1991–2000, which of course was verified by my medical appeal tribunal in 2004.

The dorsal root ganglion (DRG) is an exception to the otherwise restricted permeability between blood and nervous tissue, much like the blood-brain barrier. The DRG exhibits high permeability, which could be of significant clinical relevance because this makes it vulnerable to both high and low molecular weight, including neurotoxic substances/metabolites from drugs and chemical toxic exposures which can include neuropathies. More information can be found on the National Centre for Biotechnology Information (NCBI) website.

Work has been going on for years in Australia to examine excretion of chemicals, which could be abnormal products of metabolism in patients with ME–CFS. In fact, the researchers found the chemical structure is similar to that of a neuroactive drug, which inhibits one of the brain receptors and alters neurotransmitter activity and the HPA axis (Hypothalamic Pituitary Adrenal axis), which verifies some of the research work undertaken by Dr Behan in which he found a highly upregulated HPA axis in ME sufferers and sheep dippers. The Australian research also found some similarities with N methyl pyrrolidone (a solvent commonly used in the pesticide and pharmaceutical industries), which has been independently reported as producing symptoms similar to ME–CFS following accidental exposure. The researchers consider that these data do not suggest a psychological cause for ME–CFS.

On a personal level, in a casual conversation with my pharmacist, I asked what his professional opinion was on the use of N methyl pyrrolidone. He suggested it could cause genetic abnormalities.

In May 2021 (with seemingly magical timing) Stephanie Seneff Ph.D published the highly acclaimed book *Toxic Legacy* in which she cites lots of scientific research showing the dangers of the world's biggest-selling herbicide, Roundup (amongst other trade names), and the active ingredient glyphosate—the one I was given to use in my job. The book shows there are other probable damaging consequences, e.g. neurological and genetic effects, as well as non-Hodgkin's lymphoma, which was also reported by Carey Gillam in her brilliant, groundbreaking book *Whitewash*. (As far back as 1994 a report appeared in the *Daily Mail* saying the EU were reviewing glyphosate over growing fears of its safety.)

Toxic Legacy cites research from the Texas Health Science Center in San Antonio that showed women with my condition—multiple chemical sensitivities, which most sufferers have to a lesser or larger degree—have three times the risk of having a child with autism as well as other neurological disorders. These children are also more prone to allergies. The study also found that having MCS (multiple chemical sensitivity) usually reflects excessive lifetime exposure to toxic chemicals.

So there we have it: proof emerging at last after thirty years of suffering, and being told you are a hypochondriac or an all-in-the-mind merchant. Meanwhile brain diseases and cancers are massively on the increase. The biggest killer of children under fourteen is cancer.

I believe the genetic link is proven when one considers my condition, that of my niece Phillipa, who has ME–CFS and MCS, her daughter Rhianna, who has autism, and her son Brandon with ADHD.

Research shows damage to the hippocampus, the part of the brain responsible for forming and storing memories and is associated with learning and emotions. No wonder I couldn't perform at school; I couldn't remember what I had done the day before! And it may also account for my emotional standoffishness mixed with outbursts of anger, and at times rage. I see it as a smoking gun called "chemical-related neurodevelopment interference".

Some of the powers that be have helped to cover up these dangers for decades (remember tobacco?). In the past it was mainly some working class jobs that would have put you at risk. Not anymore. Exposure is pretty much unavoidable, especially from March to October, and as I've said many times to medics with closed minds: 'There is no Planet Janet to escape to.'

Despite the hope that came with reiki, at seventy years of age (as of 2020) I find it hard to be optimistic about the future. While I am on a relatively even keel at present, one day I may face a serious illness, a nightmare scenario that may necessitate taking drugs, which I believe would finish me off.

Reiki saved me when I was ill, and hopefully it will save me when the end is close.

I shall finish by saying a big thank you to my ex-partner Eileen. We stayed together until February 2018 when she left to be closer to her family in Oswaldtwistle. We remained friends after we split up and still keep in touch, so there is no animosity between us. She comes to my place every six weeks or so for a meal. I admire how she soldiered on after being diagnosed with MS aged thirty-two. After her mother passed and she lost the ability to drive, I could see she was getting depressed because she couldn't get out of the house too easily.

I always ask for the greatest good for both her and me. I believe that it is for Eileen's greatest good to be living on her own. She's near her son and grandson who she can now see regularly, and I'm glad that her health is stable.

People might wonder, *How and why does he keep in touch with someone who walked out on him*? Reiki taught me that being bitter will stop you getting better. Reiki works for the greatest good, so sometimes the power is not for you personally. Even when I was sleeping on the couch and she was sleeping in the bed, I would send Eileen an absent healing twice a week—for her greatest good. We both suffered together for over thirty years, so to get as far as we did was a miracle. Reiki eased the path for us to live separate lives and for both of us to be happier. After she left, even though I was upset, I realised that that was the greatest good in the long run.

I also believe we came into this world with a pre-ordained plan. Everything strongly points to MS and ME being caused by chemicals. I think we came to prove a point about suffering, finding a way and seeing it through, and seeing the spiritual healing it can bring.

I certainly don't blame Eileen for leaving; she had a lot to put up with. I realise now that no one could have coped with me and my condition—not just the life changes but also missing out on all the normal things that make a life: no socialising or holidays, no cinemas or restaurants, only two hours of heating on in the winter, all these restrictions must have driven her crazy. I struggled to cope with it myself sometimes.

I never knew how bad I was going to feel each morning when I woke up, except that two days of every week I would be either detoxifying or toxed up, bedbound and in a foul mood, like a junkie without a fix. Indeed, I call everyone in my situation 'environmental junkies'. We are at the mercy of whatever chemicals we are exposed to (remember, evidence is also being linked to MS). She used to tell me that the smell from the chemical plant she worked at was so obnoxious that it was unbearable.

So thank you, Eileen, for being a brave soldier for so long. I could not have recovered from my hip fracture in 2012 or made it this far without your twice weekly reiki sessions.

My mora therapist, Karen Barlow, says I am a natural born fighter. I don't know about that. But hopefully this book will change some hearts and minds and help get better treatment for people with MS–CFS, end the discrimination against us, and maybe inspire some people with ME and others to find their own natural path to improving their health and avoid toxing themselves up unnecessarily.

Love and light to all,
Brian

They broke my heart, my body and sometimes my mind, but they couldn't break my spirit.

BIBLIOGRAPHY

Detoxify or Die, Dr Sherry Rogers

Stop the 21st Century Killing You, Dr Paula Baillie-Hamilton

Diagnosis and Treatment of Chronic Fatigue Syndrome and Myalgic Encephalitis Second Edition: it's mitochondria, not hypochondria, Sarah Myhill

Whitewash: The story of a Weedkiller, Cancer and the Corruption of Science, Carey Gillam

Vibrational Medicine, Richard Gerber, MD

Infinite Mind: Science of the Human Vibrations of Consciousness, Valerie V Hunt

Biochemical Individuality: Basis for the Genetotrophic Concept, Roger J Williams, PhD

Staying Alive in Toxic Times: A Seasonal Guide to Lifelong Health, Dr Jenny Goodman

Proof of Heaven: A neurosurgeon's journey into the afterlife, Dr Eben Alexander

M.E., Dr Ann Macintyre

Skewed, Martin J Walker

Not All in the Mind, Dr Richard Mackarness

Chemical Victims, Dr Richard Mackarness

CFS: A Delayed Reaction to Chronic Low Dose of Exposure, 1996, Professor Peter Behan

Toxic Legacy: How the weedkiller glyphosate is destroying our health and the environment, 2021, Stephanie Seneff, Ph.D

Toxic Induced Loss of Tolerance, Claudia Miller

Silent Spring, Rachel Carson

The Chemical Age, Frank A. von Hippel

Reiki for Life, Penelope Quest

The Reiki Manual, Penelope Quest & Kathy Roberts

Psychic Discoveries: The Iron Curtain Lifted, Sheila Ostrander & Lynn Schroeder

REFERENCES

Chronic fatigue syndrome as a delayed reaction to low dose organophosphate exposure, article in *Journal of Nutritional and Environmental Medicine*, 1997; pp.341–350, P.O. Behan

Cognitive function following exposure to contaminated air on commercial aircraft: A case series of 27 pilots seen for clinical purposes, article in *Journal of Nutritional and Environmental Medicine*, 2009, vol 17, issue 2; pp. 111–126, Sarah Mackenzie Ross

www.angelfleet.net You can make flying safer for yourself by obtaining a Sky Mask.

ACKNOWLEDGEMENTS

My thanks go to

Reflexologist Emily Doherty who treated me 2017–2019. We had a real connection before she moved to Majorca.

Mora therapist Karen Barlow whose skills have been invaluable, especially when my sensitivities have risen due to further chemical exposure.

Geraldine Coobhan, reiki master, who sends me regular distant reiki healings. Whenever I'm in a bad state she has been very helpful.

Geraldine Murray: Dublin's loss was Manchester's gain.

Mira Bela, go to reikidivinemaster@gmail.com

I would also like to thank Alan Whelan for his invaluable help in the writing of this book. Go to www.alanwhelan.co.uk for more.

Lightning Source UK Ltd.
Milton Keynes UK
UKHW040835250522
403501UK00003B/186

9 781916 081963